CLASSICAL
T'AI CHI
SWORD

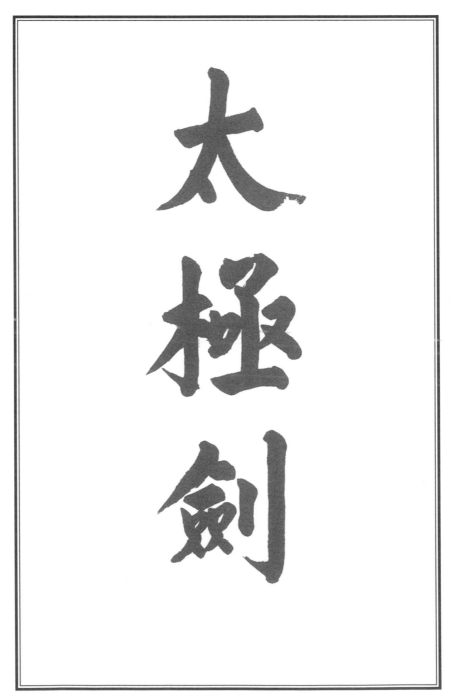

太極劍

T'AI CHI SWORD

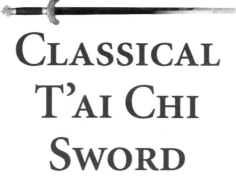

CLASSICAL T'AI CHI SWORD

TOYO & PETRA KOBAYASHI

CONTRIBUTIONS BY CHIANG TAO CHI

TUTTLE PUBLISHING
Tokyo · Rutland, Vermont · Singapore

Originally published as *Die Schwertkunst des T'ai Chi Ch'uan*, Copyright © 1995 Heinrich Hugendubel Verlag

Published by Tuttle Publishing, an imprint of Periplus Editions (HK) Ltd., with editorial offices at 364 Innovation Drive, North Clarendon, Vermont 05759 U.S.A.

Translated and revised, 2002: Susan Rae Polzer and the author.

Library of Congress Cataloging-in-Publication Data

Kobayashi, Toyo.
   [Schwertkunst des T'ai Chi Chuan. English]
   Classical t'ai chi sword / Toyo & Petra Kobayashi; contributions by Chiang Tao Chi.
     p. cm.
   ISBN 0-08048-3448-2 (pbk.)
   1. Swordplay—China. 2. Tai chi. I. Kobayashi, Petra. II. Chi, Chiang Tao, 1920-1994.
III. Title.

GV1150 .K63 2003

613.7'148—dc21   2002075655

ISBN-10: 0-8048-3448-2
ISBN-13: 978-0-8048-3448-3

Distributed by

North America,
Latin America & Europe
Tuttle Publishing
364 Innovation Drive
North Clarendon, VT 05759-9436 U.S.A.
Tel: 1 (802) 773-8930
Fax: 1 (802) 773-6993
info@tuttlepublishing.com
www.tuttlepublishing.com

Asia Pacific
Berkeley Books Pte. Ltd.
61 Tai Seng Avenue
Singapore 534167
Tel: (65) 6280-1330
Fax: (65) 6280-6290
inquiries@periplus.com.sg
www.periplus.com

Japan
Tuttle Publishing
Yaekari Building, 3rd Floor
5-4-12 Osaki
Shinagawa-ku
Tokyo 141 0032
Tel: (81) 3 5437-0171
Fax: (81) 3 5437-0755
tuttle-sales@gol.com

First edition
10 09 08 07   10 9 8 7 6 5 4 3
Design by Linda Carey
Printed in Singapore

TUTTLE PUBLISHING® is a registered trademark of Tuttle Publishing,
a division of Periplus Editions (HK) Ltd.

CONTENTS

ACKNOWLEDGMENTS

Our special thanks go to Swantje Autrum-Mulzer for the photographs; Yen Shih, Janni Endriss, and Lin De Huei for the translation from the Chinese; Master Ma Chang Xun for the calligraphy; the painter Dito for the drawings; Tathata Kobayashi for the portrayal of the partner exercises; Beatrix Schumacher for her collaboration; and Susan Rae Polzer for the English translation and help with the revision.

Foreword

I felt honored when Petra and Toyo Kobayashi asked me to write the foreword for this brilliantly conceived and well-organized book on T'ai Chi sword. It is truly useful and informative for all students of T'ai Chi, regardless of the style or form of practice. The instructive photos are ingeniously diagrammed and easy to follow, making the sword forms easy to learn. And the text leads the reader step-by-step through the form, clearly explaining the underlying principles.

This book is a rewarding instructional and educational experience, and I am comfortable recommending it also to martial artists of all other disciplines. It is well known that many top athletes develop proficiency in a second sport as a way of improving their skills. Those who train with weapons—especially sticks, sabers, and poles—will find this book immensely valuable. I encourage everyone to discover the lessons this ancient form has to offer. Sword adds a dynamic dimension to one's training. This book helps one achieve right practice so student and sword become completely harmonized.

Petra and Toyo are well-known throughout Europe as a result of spending the last thirty years spreading the values of classical T'ai Chi through their teaching and publications. Throughout human history, one of the most difficult and challenging tasks is that of the cultural interpreter. Petra and Toyo have become cultural bridges and ambassadors of this ancient art. This is their first book to be translated into English, and I wish it great success. We can all benefit from reading it and putting the principles into practice.

Mondo Secter, PhD on "The Architectonics of Culture," (2003). Also author of I Ching Clarified *(1993) republished as* The I Ching Handbook *(2002); and co-author of* Passionate Zen Cooking: the Art of New Japanese-Western Cuisine, *with spouse, Ari Tomita (2003).*

Preface

In T'ai Chi Ch'uan, as in other Chinese martial arts, special exercises have developed, using a sword, a saber, or a staff. The most significant exercises among these are those with the sword, which form an important art.

The key characteristic of T'ai Chi Ch'uan is the alignment of three viewpoints: self-defense, health, and meditation. This is also true for the art of the sword. It is not only a method for protecting oneself but also a comprehensive exercise for good health and meditation while in motion.

Until now, there has been little information in the West about the art of the T'ai Chi[1] sword. The encouragement to write this book comes from our T'ai Chi teacher, Dr. Chiang Tao Chi, who was one of the leading students of Cheng Man-Ching in Taiwan and is also a master of the sword.[2] His knowledge and experience were an important influence on us.

Dr. Chi retired from teaching in 1990 and advised my husband, Toyo Kobayashi, and me to study with T'ai Chi sword masters in China. From master Fu Zhong-Wen,[3] we learned the entire sword form of his teacher, Yang Cheng-Fu.[4] We also worked with sword masters in Shanghai and Peking whose backgrounds were in the Chen style and the Wu style. These experiences convinced us that the sword form and the thirteen sword techniques depicted in this book are at the center of the classical T'ai Chi sword as it is known today.

The sword form described in this book is as Dr. Chi taught it. Dr. Chi himself contributed some of the chapters: "A Brief History of the Chinese Sword," "Anecdote," and "The T'ai Chi Sword."

Since the sword art is based upon the same principles as the other exercises in T'ai Chi Ch'uan, the background information that is already available in the T'ai Chi literature now in circulation applies here as well. My husband and I have published three other T'ai Chi books, currently available only in German. The aspects of T'ai Chi Ch'uan that are particularly important in understanding the T'ai Chi sword will be discussed again in this volume.

A special concern of mine was to reveal the history of the T'ai Chi sword. It didn't seem to me to be sufficient to simply repeat the usual explanation from T'ai Chi literature, which states that the sword art evolved from T'ai Chi Ch'uan. Investigation into the subject has made it possible to describe the history more exactly.

It is not only the advanced T'ai Chi student who can learn sword. T'ai Chi sword is known in China as an independent path of exercise that doesn't necessarily require knowledge of the other forms of T'ai Chi Ch'uan.

---

[1] Ta'i Chi is the common abbreviation for T'ai Chi Ch'uan.
[2] Please note that the Chinese written character for *sword* means the object, the exercise, and the art. This all-inclusive meaning of the single word *sword* has been taken over in the West from the Chinese. In this book, you will also frequently find the use of the word *sword* with this Chinese meaning.
[3] See the glossary on pages 171–74.
[4] ibid.

Just like the other T'ai Chi Ch'uan exercises, the sword is geared toward the development and application of the inner energy, ch'i. The application of this energy shows us possibilities in sword fighting that go beyond what we in the West know or can imagine.

Classical T'ai Chi sword deserves the same level of interest and the same acceptance that the other forms of T'ai Chi Ch'uan have already received. Through the information presented here, we would like to contribute to the cultivation and preservation of this highly refined art in the West.

Petra Kobayashi

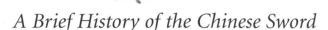

A Brief History of the Chinese Sword

Swords were already being produced in China in the third millennium B.C. It is said that the legendary ruler, Huang-Ti,[1] was forging bronze[2] swords by this time from Shou Shan copper.

Later, during the period of the Chou Dynasty (1123–255 B.C.) and during the period of the Warring States (403–221 B.C.), iron swords were produced in great numbers in the feudal states. Those of the Cheng, Wu, and Yueh dynasties were particularly outstanding. Among the swords, which varied greatly in form and size, were those that were famous for the distinct way in which they were forged and their exceptional sharpness. They were highly valued and passed on from generation to generation. Fights were frequently fought in order to obtain ownership of one of them. It wasn't unusual for a sword fighter to sacrifice his entire possessions and land, or even his life, for such a sword. The names, manufacturers, and owners of the famous swords over hundreds of years are listed, for example:

NAME OF THE SWORD	DYNASTY	OWNER	SMITHY
CHÜEH	CHOU	TAI KUNG	—
KAN CHIANG	WU	HO LÜ	KAN CHIANG MO HSIEH
CHU CHÜEH	YUEH	KING OF YUEH	OU YEH TZU

It is assumed that the craft of swordsmithing, which flourished greatly during this period due to large demand, experienced a recession in the third century B.C.

In 221 B.C., Ying Chen of the Ch'in Dynasty became the first emperor of China. During his reign, he ordered that all weapons possessed by the civilian population were to be collected and melted down.

After the fall of the Ch'in Dynasty and the rise of the Han Dynasty, the craft of swordsmithing returned to a significant portion of its original size, even though it couldn't recapture the glory of the past.

---

[1] The transcription used here is commonly found in English language T'ai Chi literature. It is derived from the earlier official language, Cantonese, and is used by expatriate Chinese in Southeast Asia and Taiwan, and in the West. The Pinjin transcription, which is promoted by the present Chinese government, developed from the Han Chinese. T'ai Chi Ch'uan is called Taijiquan, Tao is called Dao, I Ching (I Ging) is called Yiying, Chi Kung is called Qigong, and so on.

[2] Bronze is composed of 80 percent copper and 20 percent tin.

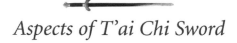

Aspects of T'ai Chi Sword

The sword form represents the heart of the art of T'ai Chi sword. The classical sword form is composed of fifty basic positions and the transitions connecting them together. Individual positions are sometimes repeated. The positions usually have pretty, picturesque names such as "The Swallow Takes Water" or "Embrace the Moon." These descriptions contain no hidden meaning, but elegantly describe the shape and nature of the movement.

The positions and the transitions contain the so-called 13[3] Sword Techniques (see "The 13 Techniques" section). Their organization and application is based upon the same principles as the sword form in general and all other T'ai Chi exercises. The use of the techniques, therefore, is not to be thought of in isolation or as being designed only for their effectiveness in sword fighting.

Practicing the techniques with a partner is an important part of the study of T'ai Chi sword. However, the basis for improvement in the sword is the year-long practice of the sword form, which the student performs by himself. In addition to providing many positive effects, such as improving the state of one's health (see the "Practicing Sword as an Exercise for Good Health" section), this leads to the development of the inner energy, Ch'i. Through the use of this inner energy, a kind of self-defense is possible that goes way beyond the application of the sword-fighting techniques alone.

---

[3] The number 13 has a special meaning in China because many traditional exercise systems are based upon the 8 Trigrams of the *I Ching* and the teaching of the 5 elements. A Taoist exercise system, such as T'ai Chi Ch'uan, with its 13 basic postures in the short form, long form, and the 13 techniques in the sword form, indicates that it is connected with the wisdom and experience of those ancient traditions.

The History of T'ai Chi Sword

To begin with, some information should be mentioned about the history of T'ai Chi in general. T'ai Chi Ch'uan, a Taoist exercise system, has an approximately one-thousand-year-old history. The so-called basic positions and rules that determine the exercises are handed down from the legendary founders (see the Glossary). The first well-known styles[4] are the Chen style (founder Chen Wan-Ting, 1597–1664) and the Yang style, which developed out of the former (founder Yang Lu-Ch'an, 1799–1872). The styles are normally named after the surnames of their founders, and a style was frequently influenced by family traditions over several generations. Starting with the development of the Yang style, T'ai Chi Ch'uan has spread widely throughout China. (The Yang style aims to redirect T'ai Chi Ch'uan to its older Taoist principles again and emphasizes, among other things, the health aspect of T'ai Chi Ch'uan.) In the meantime, a large number of other styles have been established.

Exercising with "weapon forms," such as sword, saber, staff, and spear, in T'ai Chi Ch'uan has been recorded since the period of the Chen style. At the beginning of the Chen style, however, exercising with a sword was not a priority. It is known that Yang Lu-Ch'an, founder of the Yang style, practiced sword. There is no record, however, of how his sword form looked or, for example, what similarity it had to the sword form practiced by his grandson, Yang Cheng-Fu. What is known is that from the start, the Taoist arts of the sword influenced the sword tradition of the Yang family; the connection to the "Wu Tan sword" (see the next section) can only be documented at a later point in time.

The sword form is passed down from Yang Cheng-Fu (1883–1936), whose creation of the long form influenced the T'ai Chi Ch'uan of today more that anyhing else. It was the very first T'ai Chi sword form to be written down, by his student, Chen Wei-Ming (?–1960) in the book, *The T'ai Chi Sword Fight*.[5] Although this is not a very extensive book, it contains a description of the motions, photographs of the positions, and their names in performance. From what Chen Wei-Ming writes, Yang Cheng-Fu taught no special application of the sword techniques. He was known to use the "sticking energy" for sword fighting.[6]

This explains why Chen Wei-Ming sought a teacher who could instruct him in the application of the sword techniques. As he describes it in his book, he found that teacher in Li Chin-Lin (1860–1920), a man who was in close contact with the Yang family and who later turned out to have a decisive influence on the emergence of the present T'ai Chi sword. Li Chin-Lin, a general and the intermittent governor of the Hopei Province, was

---

[4] We describe a style as a specific development in T'ai Chi Ch'uan on the basis of the same principles.
[5] This is the original Chinese title translated into English.
[6] We know from various sources that exercising "with empty hands" was a priority for Yang Cheng-Fu, who only taught sword to a limited extent.

known in his time as one of the best sword fighters in China. He practiced the old art of the Taoist "Wu Tan sword." His teacher, Chen Shih-Chüen, continued this art into the twelfth generation.[7] The creation of Wu Tan sword is attributed to the Taoist master Chang San-Feng, who is also considered one of the founders of T'ai Chi Ch'uan (Chang San-Feng lived in the period of the Sung Dynasty, 1127–1279, on Wu Tan Mountain). This already indicates the close connection between the Wu Tan art of the sword and T'ai Chi Ch'uan.

General Li promoted the art of the sword and demonstrated it in many places. Among the places he traveled to was Japan. Apparently T'ai Chi Ch'uan was of great importance to him (see the "Anecdote" section). His T'ai Chi teacher was Yang Pan-Hou (1837–1892, second generation of the Yang family), who was a well-known personality in the Yang style. In addition, as Fu Zhong-Wen has informed us,[8] not only was Li a close friend of Yang Cheng-Fu but they were also blood brothers. One can imagine that they exchanged information about T'ai Chi Ch'uan and the art of the sword. As will later be described, their sword forms are similar in their essential aspects.

Under the influence of T'ai Chi Ch'uan, Li founded a new, or modern, Wu Tan sword. It was so closely related to T'ai Chi Ch'uan that it continued under the name "The T'ai Chi sword."[9] In it, elements of the Wu Tan sword are joined with T'ai Chi Ch'uan and with the sword tradition of the Yang family. Its 13 Techniques (see "The 13 Techniques" section) are supposed to have been derived from the Wu Tan sword techniques.

Until that time, practicing with a sword had only occurred in accompaniment with other T'ai Chi exercises; it now took the form of a separate discipline. From that time on, it became popular to practice exclusively with the sword.

The art of the sword defined here also had an influence, beyond the Yang style, on the sword in other T'ai Chi styles. Today, these styles practice similar sword forms, with the characteristic features of their own style. In Yang Cheng-Fu's circle of students, his sword form continues to be taught without reference to the 13 Techniques; therefore, his students' sword books, for example, don't go into details about the techniques.

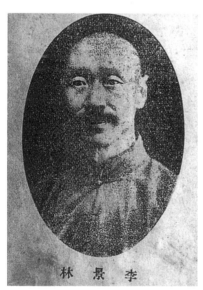

林景李

Li Chin-Lin

---

[7] Matsuda. *Chinese Martial Arts*, page 106, only available in the Japanese edition.
[8] See the glossary on pages 171–74.
[9] Matsuda. *Chinese Martial Arts*, page 106.

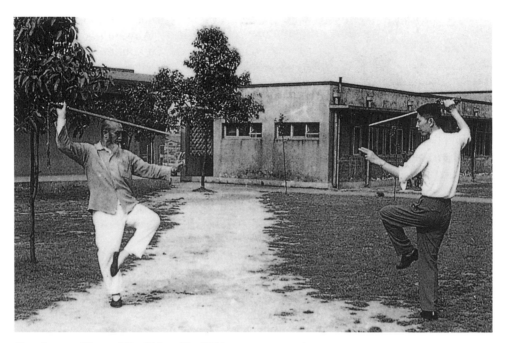
Sword master Hsu and Dr. Chiang Tao Chi in a partner exercise

The T'ai Chi sword in the Cheng Man-Ch'ing tradition also goes back to Yang Cheng-Fu. Cheng Man-Ch'ing,[10] whose short form decisively influenced T'ai Chi Ch'uan in the West, was a principal student of Yang Cheng-Fu, from whom he learned the sword form.

Dr. Chiang Tao Chi[11] studied sword with Cheng Man-Ch'ing in Taiwan. When Cheng Man-Ch'ing left for America, Dr. Chi worked with the sword master Hsu.[12] Hsu studied, among others, in the General Li tradition. He also learned the art of "San T'sai sword"[13] from Sun Lu-Tang.[14]

[10-14] See the glossary on pages 171–74.

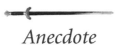

Anecdote

Li Chin-Lin, famous as the best sword fighter in China and a former governor of the Hopei Province, served in his younger years as a regimental commander.

He was already a master of the martial arts at this time and was proud and confident of his ability.

One day he found himself in the company of some friends who convinced him to show them some of his martial arts. By chance, he saw an old man among the spectators who was shaking his head in amusement. Surprised and curious, Li went to him and said: "If I am not mistaken, sir, you are an expert in this area." "Thank you, but you flatter me," answered the old man. At Li's request, he demonstrated the T'ai Chi Ch'uan form in its full length. All the movements were connected together so effortlessly that Li was truly delighted.

"Excuse me, sir, are you equally good in the sword?" asked Li.

"Not quite," answered the old man, "but you can nevertheless pull your sword; I shall try to defend myself with the stem of my tobacco pipe.[15] So, let's try it."

When everything was ready, Li attacked with his sword in his hand. No sooner had he flicked his sword forward but the pipe of the old man was already sticking to it. However much he tried, his attempts to free himself were to no avail.

Now that he recognized that his opponent was considerably superior to him, he retreated and requested the old man to instruct him.

***

From what we know, Li learned from Yang Pan-Hou, the oldest son of Yang Lu-Ch'an, the founder of the Yang style, and from Chen Shih-Chüen and Sung Wei-I, both exceptional sword fighters.

The old man in the story was supposedly Yang Pan-Hou.

---

[15] Such a pipe had a stem that was several feet long and was preferred by the country folk in China.

The Taoist Background

Exercises for health, meditation, and self-defense were practiced in China long before our modern era. This led to a rich knowledge of the inherent laws that underlie the existence of man and life. Characteristic of the Taoist[16] exercises is the reference to the subtle energy realm in the nature of human beings. In this realm, which is built out of subtle, or inner, energy (see the "Energy" section), are the energy centers (*tan t'iens*[17]) and the pathways of the energy (meridians[18]). From a Taoist point of view, this area connects the physical with the psychic and the mental. The subtle energy realm, also referred to as the "subtle energy body," shows a spiritual structure. One can have an affect on it through exercises that are connected with certain body postures, movement, breathing, relaxation, and mental concentration, among others. The energy itself and the centers can be developed; pathways of energy can be activated, that is, opened;[19] and so on.

T'ai Chi Ch'uan, as a Taoist exercise system, contains exercises geared toward that effect. Developments in the subtle energy body have a positive effect on one's physical, psychic, and mental health. T'ai Chi practice, as they say, makes the "true nature" of human beings accessible and leads to the highest goal of Taoism: the oneness with the Tao. Developments in the subtle energy realm are also a preliminary for self-defense in the T'ai Chi Ch'uan sense. This explains the simultaneous relationships in T'ai Chi Ch'uan of the three aspects of health, meditation, and self-defense. The Taoist background of T'ai Chi Ch'uan reveals itself in the classical treatises[20] associated with it. The principles set down within these treatises (see the next section) describe rules that determine the structure and implementation of the exercises. They relate to the contents and the values that have a central importance in Taoist spirituality: development of the center (centering), reference to the essential, the Yin-Yang principle, naturalness, following, releasing (letting go), withdrawing oneself, unintentional action, and so on. It is fascinating how in T'ai Chi Ch'uan, as in classical T'ai Chi sword, these values have entered the process of exercising in motion. Their interplay strengthens the positive effects that are associated with each individual maxim. The principles that determine the outer structure and the implementation of the exercises are always designed with a view to the effectiveness of the exercise on internal development too.

---

[16] In Taoism, the lesson of Tao, the Nameless, the Absolute, is usually attributed to Laotse (circa 600 B.C.). Laotse's treatise, the *Tao Te Ching* is considered the fundamental work in Taoism.

[17] The most important centers in the Taoist tradition are the lower, middle, and upper tan t'iens. The orientation on the physical body for the lower tan t'ien is located below the navel, the middle tan t'ien at the level of the solar plexus, the upper tan t'ien in the upper part of the head. Corresponding to the tan t'iens are the chakras in the Indian traditions.

[18] The meridian system corresponds to the organs of the human body. The thousand-year-old Chinese acupuncture system works with them.

[19] Other Chinese exercise systems known in the West that effect the subtle energy realm, as T'ai Chi Ch'uan does, are the exercises for health in the Chi Kung and Taoist meditation methods, designed to open the "Heavenly Circles."

[20] See the glossary on pages 171–74.

Important Principles of T'ai Chi Ch'uan[21]

relax - release (let go) - sink

root - yield - follow - join (connect)

lively - light - natural

even - slow - continuous

directed - balanced

movement from the center

curved movement

upright-straightening from within

not going to the extreme

full and empty

open and close

keeping to the essentials

deep breathing

meditative state of mind

[21] See the glossary on pages 171–74.

Practicing Sword as an Exercise for Good Health

The sword form, like all exercises in T'ai Chi Ch'uan, has a comprehensive effect upon physical, psychic, and mental health.[22] Here are some examples:

In lifting, sinking, forward, and backward movement, and in the circularity of many movements, the joints are moved easily, evenly, and gently as suits their construction. This restores the flexibility of the practitioner, that is, maintains it and leads to a general strengthening of the body. The connection between the healing and the prevention of various diseases in the movement system of the body is thus shown.

Leading the movement of the body and the sword from the hip area straightens the spine and massages and strengthens the inner organs.

Moving in the characteristic way of T'ai Chi Ch'uan relaxes, calms, and promotes the functions of the nervous system.

The increased ability to relax that results from exercising with the sword is connected with deeper breathing, which takes the strain off the heart, improves the use of the lung capacity, and, therefore, the metabolic and other functions.

The development of the subtle, or inner, energy (see the "Energy" section) that results from practicing supports and strengthens the functions of the meridian system. This is also significant for psychic and mental health. It stabilizes and harmonizes the human being.

---

[22] Nowadays, many people in China practice it for health reasons alone.

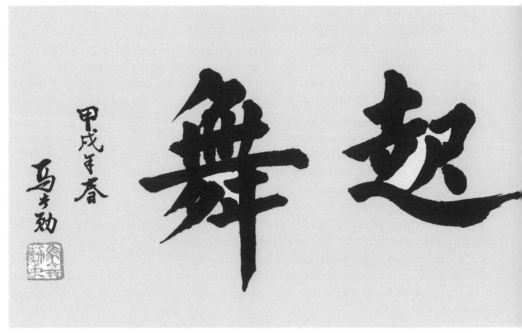

Early in the morning, with the cock's first crow, I begin my exercising.

The sword is practiced with a meditative attitude of mind. As in the short and the long forms, two methods are commonly used. One way is the concentration on the lower tan t'ien, which is held there during the entire form. This method is practiced, for example, in the Cheng Man-Ching tradition. The other way relies on exercising with the utmost attention and is comparable to Shikantaza in Zen Buddhist meditation. This technique is used, among others, by the Yang family and their followers, including master Fu Zhong-Wen. Both methods lead to the state of non-thinking (empty mind). Naturally, it takes many years of practicing to become accomplished in each of these methods.

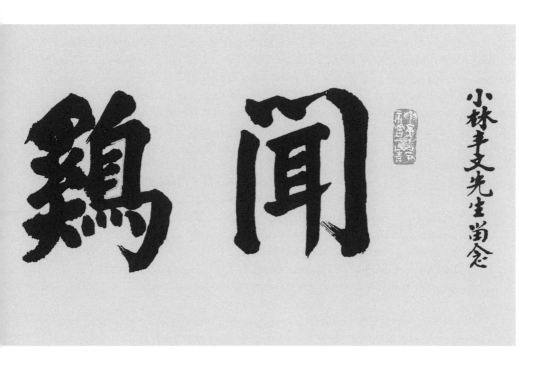

Understandably, a meditative state of mind is difficult to achieve in the beginning. Frequently, thoughts will arise in the first years of practicing the forms, as they do in sitting meditation. With growing relaxation and the ability to sink the energy, the state of non-thinking increases and prevails. This is an indication that the student has advanced on his or her way.

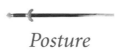

Posture

The posture of the body used for practicing the sword is the same as the one used for the short and the long forms. As one says in T'ai Chi, the posture should be in harmony with the forces of heaven and earth.[23] The subtle energy (also called cosmic energy) is in alignment with these forces. The rising ch'i is called the "Heaven Ch'i" and the sinking ch'i is called the "Earth Ch'i." The action of these two complementary forces is clearly experienced in advanced practice. In harmony with the rising of the ch'i, the body follows by straightening from within, which, among other things, makes it possible to easily and effortlessly hold the torso. Along with the sinking of the ch'i, balance and "rooting" take place, which is very important in T'ai Chi Ch'uan.

In the center of the posture is the torso. Some important rules concerning it are:

- The chin is somewhat pulled in to straighten the cervical vertebrae.
- The chest is relaxed.
- The shoulders are released and hang down.
- The hips and the lower back are relaxed.
- The spine is held straight and vertical.[24]

The position of the limbs follows and agrees with the position of the torso: bending the knees during the exercises allows the release of the lower back; the arms are usually held slightly rounded and, like the legs, shouldn't be completely straightened, which helps to maintain the relaxed position of the upper body.

A posture in this sense is beneficial for the development of the inner energy. From a Taoist point of view, it contributes to the harmony of human beings with themselves and the world.

---

[23] Also see *Der Weg des T'ai Chi Ch'uan* by Petra Kobayashi, currently available only in German.
[24] The same posture is used when practicing sitting meditation.

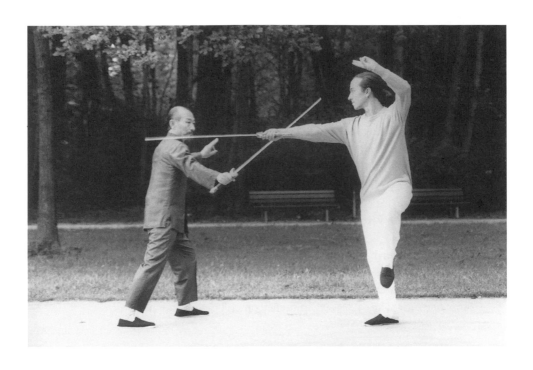

Exercises from the San T'sai Sword

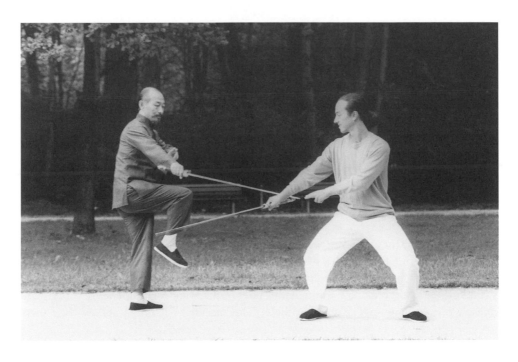

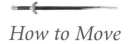

How to Move

The common characteristics of moving in T'ai Chi Ch'uan also apply in practicing the sword. The movements should be performed slowly, evenly, and in as relaxed a manner as possible.

With reference to speed, there is a slight difference in the performance of the sword form. This is explained by the "extension" of the body through the sword. The energy, ch'i, that should not only move through the body but also into the sword, must cover an appropriately longer path than in the short or the long form (empty hands). Therefore, a somewhat faster performance in the first years of practicing apparently makes it easier to move the ch'i into the sword. With increased development of the ch'i, slower movement can work equally well.

In the sword form, movement is also directed; lively; and up to the end of the positions and the transitions, polarized through "open and close." "Close" refers to collecting the energy. "Open" relates to directing the energy outward.

How one moves has a decisive influence on ch'i development.

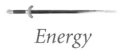

Energy

Knowledge about energy has been transmitted from ancient times in the Taoist traditions. The subtle energy, ch'i,[25] is understood to maintain the animate and inanimate nature. Existing everywhere and permeating everything, it is also called the life force, big, cosmic, or inner energy. It is approachable through a refined sensitivity (which develops by practicing T'ai Chi Ch'uan), and it can be described. The advanced T'ai Chi student perceives it, for example, in a wide and flowing movement.

Experiences in practicing show that there are specific characteristics that are valid for the ch'i, such as the above-described sinking and rising. Ch'i can also be moved by the mind. It reacts, in addition, to the movements of the body, especially arced, light, and directed movements. First and foremost, however, ch'i is inexhaustible. That means: even in the movement of energy, as it occurs in T'ai Chi Ch'uan when shifting one's weight, energy is still present in the so-called "empty."

In T'ai Chi Ch'uan, much of the practice is connected with the basic existing big ch'i. The outer form of the positions and how one moves are so constructed as to stimulate the energy to flow through the body. This wide floating energy movement doesn't use the pathways of the meridians. The meridians naturally follow their own

---

[25] In Indian Yoga "prana," in Japanese "ki."

directions in a fixed system designed to maintain the functions of the physical body. Although the energy movement doesn't use the meridians, it still helps to activate and strengthen their functions. The repetition of the movement of the ch'i over many years plays a decisive role in what is known in T'ai Chi Ch'uan as ch'i development.

Ch'i Development

Ch'i development begins with the very first step that one takes in T'ai Chi. It is a complex process in which a large number of additional factors play a role; for example, the "movement" of energy, breathing, relaxation, releasing, body posture, and mental attentiveness.

The significance of the term ch'i development is the growth of energy. This has various effects:

- It is beneficial to the functional strength of the meridians.
- Through the activation of the energy centers and the opening of the meridians, it leads to spiritual development and prepares one for spiritual experiences such as enlightenment.
- The developed ch'i can be used in self-defense. It shows qualities that in T'ai Chi are understood to be separate energies—listening, understanding, feeling, sticking, and exploding energy. All of these accompanying attributes of the developed ch'i are made accessible through practicing. (In advanced practice, the term ch'i development is filled with new meaning. It becomes clear that the ch'i development experienced by the student is not only due to his own efforts. More specifically, some of the unbelievable power of the already existing ch'i becomes gradually available to the student.)

T'ai Chi Ch'uan exercises are oriented towards setting the ch'i development on its way. If we assume that the sword form is usually learned after many years of practicing the short or the long forms, the practitioners bring their already accomplished energy development with them when practicing the sword form. If practitioners begin the sword form without previous experience in T'ai Chi Ch'uan, they must practice and develop the energy through the sword form, that is, through frequent repetition over the years in order to find the entrance to the higher art of the T'ai Chi sword.

The Movement of Energy by Practicing the Sword Form

The movement of energy through the body explained here refers to a position performed in a Bow Step (see page 43). With some variations, it is also valid for the other steps. The movement of energy through the body runs in the following way:

Forward-legs: Starting with the back foot, through the leg, following a slight arc passing through the hip area (lower tan t'ien) then downward through the leg to the front foot. (At the end of shifting forward as well as at the end of shifting backward, a slight releasing in the groin fold is used to collect the energy in the foot and the area surrounding it (center equilibrium). This acts as a spring, helping to mobilize one's energy effortlessly upward into the next movement.

Forward-torso, arms, and sword: When the energy has reached the lower tan t'ien area, it separates. One part moves, as already described, into the front leg, the other part continues upward through the torso and the arms into the, at times, active part of the blade. This also refers to horizontal and downward movement of the sword.

Backward: The backward movement is the reverse of that described above. The energy from the sword, arms, and upper torso sinks into the lower tan t'ien, helping with the collection of energy there. This combines with the energy from the front leg. Together they sink into the back foot (center equilibrium).

Additional Points:

- Although the time for collecting the energy in the lower tan t'ien seems to be rather short in the sword form, it is constantly recurring, as in the short and long forms, according to the yin-yang principle.
- In order to move the energy into the sword, the movement must be slightly accelerated. The movement of the energy into the sword finger is subordinate.
- In the prescribed routes of movement, the energy "crosses" through the torso or it stays on the same side of the body.[26]
- Following the principles of T'ai Chi Ch'uan, the movement of energy through the entire sword form is directed by the center of the body. In the term "center," physical functions join with energetic functions. The hips (hip joints) and the lower tan t'ien, forming the center, guide the complex movement of the body and energy. A high-quality T'ai Chi method is oriented to bring the best results by being in harmony with natural laws and conditions.

---

[26] The crossing and direct routes of energy are the same in the sword form as they are in the short and long forms.

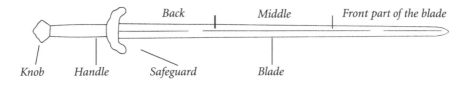

The T'ai Chi Sword

The sword used in T'ai Chi sword is commonly found in the Chinese martial arts. It is divided into the blade and the haft:

- The double-sided blade has a length of about 75 cm (29 in.) and comes to a point.
- The haft is composed of a safeguard, a handle, and a knob.

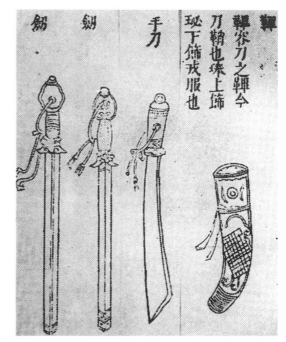

Back   *Middle*   *Front part of the blade*

Knob   *Handle*   *Safeguard*   *Blade*

The "active" (mostly turned away from the body) side of the blade of the sword is called "yang," the other side is correspondingly called "yin."

In practicing the T'ai Chi sword form, an unsharpened metal practice sword or a wooden sword is usually used. For partner exercises, it is advisable to use a wooden sword. If the student is of shorter stature, a somewhat shorter sword can be chosen.

You can make a simple wooden sword by yourself from this drawing. Metal T'ai Chi swords can be found in budo shops (martial arts specialists). Pay special attention to making sure that the sword is well made and that the blade is stable.

From an old sword book

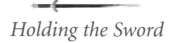

Holding the Sword

At the start of the sword form, the sword is held in the left hand; the middle finger, ring finger, little finger, and thumb hold the guard; the forefinger lies on the hilt (see diagram 1).

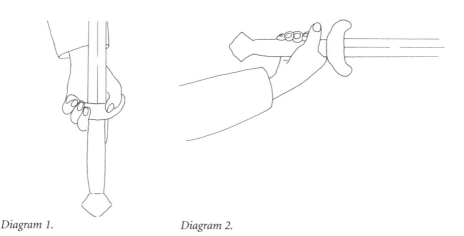

Diagram 1.   *Diagram 2.*

In the course of the form, after "Circling the Moon Three Times," the right hand holds the sword. The thumb and forefinger lie near the safeguard. As determined by the course of movement, the handle "plays" in the entire hand and lies on various parts of the palm. Even when it appears that all the fingers are holding the handle, the thumb, middle finger, and ring finger have the strongest grip and direct the movement. Note: The sword should be held safely but not too tightly in the hand.

Why the Sword Should Be Held This Way:

- Distinct coordination of the body and the sword with each other becomes possible.
- The handle can "play" in the hand. The sword can be moved lightly. Necessary changes in the movement can be performed rapidly, for example, as a reaction to an attack. (This helps to prevent "double weighting.")
- The handle can be turned or otherwise moved with the least possible bending of the wrist. Therefore, the sword can be directed in many movements from the elbow (T'ai Chi Hand). The wrist is relieved.
- The sword can be directed from the unity and from the center of the body.
- The actual weight of the sword can be incorporated into the movement.

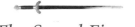

The Sword Finger

The sword finger acts, so to speak, as an extension of the arm—this can be distinctly felt by the advanced student as an "energy staff" reaching out from the fingertips.

The sword finger is held throughout the entire form by the hand that is not holding the sword. Exceptions are the series of movements during which the left hand is under the right, for example, "The Swallow Flies into the Nest" and "The Clever Cat Catches a Mouse."

Reasons for Using the Sword Finger Include the Following:

- The sword finger serves as a counterpart to the movements performed with the sword. It helps the practitioner to maintain his or her balance.
- The position of the sword finger (hand) itself can be clearly observed by the practitioner. This is important in a fight using sharp blades—in this way, injuries such as the cutting off of the hand forming the sword finger by the opponent or even by his or her own sword can be prevented.
- According to tradition, the sword finger can weaken an opponent when directed at his acupuncture points.
- With the sword finger, it is possible, in a fighting situation, to make additional movements that disorient the opponent.

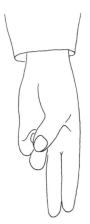

The forefinger and middle finger are extended. The upper part of the thumb lies on the fingernails of the ring finger and little finger. Ring finger, little finger, and the thumb form a circle.

The 13 Techniques[27]

1. **Ch'ou** Pull (drag)—from left to right

2. **T'ai** Take along (skim)—from right to left

3. **T'i** Lift

4. **Ke** Block

5. **Chi** Strike

6. **Tz'u** Thrust (pierce)

7. **Tien** Direct

8. **Peng** Snap (burst)

9. **Chiao** Stir (move)

10. **Ya** Press Downward

11. **Pi** Split

12. **Chieh** Intercept and attack

13. **Hsi** Clear and resolve

The following four techniques are considered basic:

Pi (split), Tz'u (thrust), Ke (block), Hsi (clear and resolve).

---

[27] In a comparison of the diverse sword forms and the techniques included in their positions, it must be remembered that even small changes in the external form and way of moving necessitate the use of different techniques.

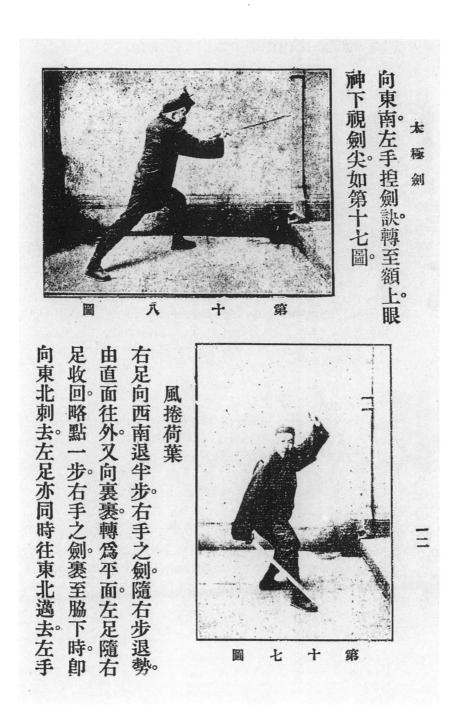

向東南。左手捏劍訣轉至額上。眼神下視劍尖如第十七圖。

第十八圖

風捲荷葉

右足向西南退半步右手之劍隨右步退勢。由直面往外又向裏裹轉為平面左足隨右足收回略點一步右手之劍裹至脅下時即向東北刺去左足亦同時往東北邁去左手

第十七圖

二

From Chen Wei-Ming's book The Tai Chi Sword Fight

The 13 Techniques in Detail[28]

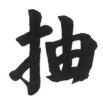

1. **Ch'ou** (Pull—from left to right):
   With the arm extended forward, pull the sword to the right.

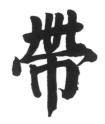

2. **T'ai** (take along or skim—from right to left):
   Move the sword from right to left in a manner that is similar to sharpening a pencil with a knife. Ch'ou and T'ai are normally combined together: After the employment of Ch'ou, the sword is immediately pulled back, and T'ai is performed in the opposite direction. T'ai can also come before Ch'ou. Ch'ou and T'ai are contained in the position, "Detain and Come Forward—Left[29] and Right."

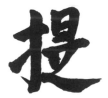

3. **T'i** (lift):
   Lift the sword upward by moving the point of the sword forward. This movement is contained in the "Small Star of the Big Dipper."

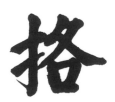

4. **Ke** (block):
   Block an attack with the lower part of the blade near the guard. This movement is contained in the positions "The Black Dragon Hits with His Tail" and "The White Tiger Hits with His Tail."

---

[28] The meaning of the techniques and their differences are not always clearly indicated in the Chinese names themselves. Translation from the Chinese is thus obviously a problem. Therefore, the various renderings in T'ai Chi literature in the West have apparently lead to the use of different designations for the same techniques. This is particularly true when the translation is only one of language, without closer knowledge of the techniques.

[29] In Chinese, left is always mentioned before right, even when, as occurs in this position, the movement performed first to the right and then to the left.

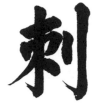
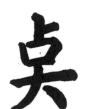
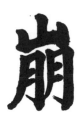
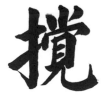

5. **Chi** (strike):

Chi is used in all the strikes, with the cutting edge of the blade aimed against the opponent from the side. This movement is contained in, for example, "The Phoenix Spreads Its Wings."

6. **Tz'u** (thrust or pierce):

Thrust the sword forward by extending your arm. This movement is contained in, for example, "The Swallow Flies into the Nest."

7. **Tien** (direct):

Tien is a small touch, a little push or scratch with the point of the sword (with the blade either standing [vertical] or lying) to startle the opponent. Tien can be used at the torso or the wrist. It is contained in the positions "Waiting for the Fish" and "The Dragonfly Touches the Water." After Tien, another technique is usually used.

8. **Peng** (snap or burst):

Turn the point of the sword in a snapping wrist movement while lifting it up from below. This movement is contained in "Lifting the Moon from the Bottom of the Sea."

9. **Chiao** (stir or move):

With the blade sticking to the opponent's sword, move it in a circle. The opponent's sword can also be pushed down, and from there the movement can continue into a thrusting one. This movement is contained in the beginning of the position "The Carp Jumps Through the Dragon Gate."

10. Ya (press downward):

With the flat of the blade, press downward on the opponent's sword. This movement is contained in "Embrace the Moon."

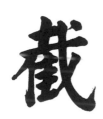

11. Pi (split):

Pi is mostly used from up to down. It is related to Tien but much larger. Generally the middle of the blade is used in Pi. If the opponent is farther away, Pi can be performed with the front part of the blade. This movement is contained in "Whirlwind Left."

12. Chieh (intercept and attack):

Chieh contains the intercepting of an assault with an immediately following attack. The blade is moved in a manner similar to a saw cutting in one direction. For example, an attack that comes first from the left and then from the upper right, moving downward, could be met with Chieh. In that way, the first attack could be countered with the flat side of the blade, and afterward the sword would be aimed from below at the opponent. Chieh is contained in "Shake Off the Dust in the Wind."

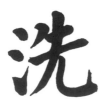

13. Hsi (clear and resolve):

Hsi represents a special use of the sword, during which sticking energy is used. Through a light, continuous touching with the blade of the sword, the opponent can be controlled, and at an appropriate moment, the sword can be directed at the opponent. This movement is contained in "The Sword Circles Like a Cartwheel— Left and Right."

The Techniques in the Sword Form Sequence

In addition to the techniques described below, individual positions can also use other techniques from the basic thirteen. The further application of the techniques becomes evident when the basic uses described here are taken to heart.

1. Awaken the Chi at the Beginning	No technique.
2. Circling the Moon Three Times	No technique.
3. Great Star of the Big Dipper	No technique, except for the preparation for the technique included in "The Swallow Takes Water."
4. The Swallow Takes Water	Follow the opponent with the sword moving upward and direct Chi (strike) against the opponent's legs or torso.
5. Detain and Come Forward—Left and Right	Using Ch'ou (pull), pull the sword to the right; if the opponent is quite close, the sword brushes the opponent's arm (or torso); afterward, guide the sword to the left and use T'ai (take along); the decisive hit usually comes with T'ai.
6. Small Star of the Big Dipper	Lift the sword upward by moving the tip of the sword forward, and direct T'i (lift) with it to the wrist of the opponent.
7. The Swallow Flies into the Nest	The technique Tz'u (thrust or pierce) is used here.
8. The Clever Cat Catches a Mouse	While standing on one leg and before the jump, Ya (press downward) is used; in the jump forward, the retreating opponent is then pursued with Tz'u (thrust or pierce).

9. The Dragonfly Touches the Water   Direct the sword with Tien (direct) to the opponent's wrist, touching the opponent lightly or strongly. This should cause the opponent to drop his sword, for example; normally another technique is used immediately after Tien.

10. The Bee Flies into the Hive   There is no technique contained in the first movement to the right. It is only the preparation for the movement to the left, following the maxim: "Before you can go to the left, you must turn to the right."

Stepping in a circle, keep the sword in the same position to protect yourself; you are inside the circle yourself and the opponent is outside; at the end of the sequence of the movements, Tz'u (thrust or pierce) is used.

11. The Phoenix Spreads Its Wings   With the upper half of the blade moving from left to right, direct Chi (strike) at the opponent's upper arm or the neck.

12. Whirlwind Left   The technique Pi (split) comes into action here; Pi is performed from up to down.

13. Small Star of the Big Dipper   T'i (lift) to the opponent's wrist.

14. Whirlwind Right   1. Variation: Use the technique Tz'u (thrust or pierce) in a downward left movement. 2. Variation: The techniques Hsi (clear and resolve) and Tien (direct) are combined. First use Hsi to yield and follow, and then continue into Tien.

15. Waiting for the Fish   The technique Tien (direct) is used.

16. Looking for the Snake in the Grass   Use Chi (strike) to the opponent's legs.

| 17. Embrace the Moon | Use the technique Ya (press downward); Ya can be used alone to stop an opponent's sword; however, Ya is usually followed by another technique, for example, Tz'u (thrust or pierce). |

| 18. The Bird Flies into the Forest to Rest | The technique Tz'u (thrust or pierce) is used here. |

| 19. The Black Dragon Hits with His Tail | Use Hsi (clear and resolve) when lowering the sword to the left; use Chi (strike) when the strike is performed to the lower right. |

| 20. The Wind Moves the Lotus | Tz'u (thrust or pierce) to the upper left. |

| 21. The Lion Shakes His Mane | The large turn contains no technique (transition); using Chieh (intercept and attack), direct the sword at the opponent's upper arm: "The Lion Shakes His Mane" is performed moving backward as if someone were approaching. |

| 22. The Tiger Puts His Head Between His Paws | Circling the arms and bringing the hands together, fitting the situation, move directly into Tz'u (thrust or pierce); Chiao (stir) and Ya (press downward) can also be used; another combination is Ya (press downward) followed by Peng (snap). |

| 23. The Wild Horse Springs over the Mountain Stream | Same application as in "The Clever Cat Catches a Mouse," only here the sword is held higher, at chest level, using Tz'u (thrust or pierce). |

| 24. Turn Around and Rein In the Horse | Use Chi (strike) throughout the entire turn or only near the end; drawing the arms in at the end of the movement collects the energy. |

| 25. Step Forward—the Compass Needle Points South | Tz'u (thrust or pierce) is used. |

26. Shake Off the Dust in the Wind	An attack, first from the left and then from the upper right downward, is met with Chieh (intercept and attack); the first attack can also be received with the flat side of the blade, as in Ke (block).
27. Send the Boat Downstream	First use Hsi (clear and resolve) in the forward direction with the sword; toward the end of the movement, use Tz'u (thrust).
28. The Shooting Star Follows the Moon	Use Pi (split) to the opponent's shoulder, for example.
29. The Heavenly Horse Flies Through the Air	Pi (split).
30. Move the Curtain	Ti (lift).
31. The Sword Circles Like a Cartwheel—Left and Right	Cartwheel left: when lowering the sword backward, first use Hsi (clear and resolve) and then Tz'u (thrust or pierce). Using only Hsi or the first part of Chieh is also possible; lifting the sword is a transition. Cartwheel right: perform Tz'u (thrust or pierce) when lowering the sword backward; afterward, when the sword comes forward utilizing more energy, use Pi (split), or utilizing less energy use Tien (direct).
32. The Mythical Bird Spreads One Wing	Chi (strike).
33. Lifting the Moon from the Bottom of the Sea	During the first forward movement of the sword, direct the forward section of the blade to the opponent's legs using Chi (strike); toward the end of the movement use Peng (snap) from below to the opponent's wrist.

34. Embrace the Moon	Use Ya (press downward) with a flat-lying blade; at the same time, raise the tip of the sword.
35. The Demon Looks into the Water	Tz'u (thrust or pierce) downward; lifting the leg intensifies the thrust here. This movement can be applied against martial artists who perform their movements close to the floor.
36. The Rhinoceros Looks at the Moon	Use Ke (block) when the sword is drawn to the left.
37. Shoot the Swallow	No technique, serves as preparation and collection of energy.
38. The White Monkey Offers Fruit	Tz'u (thrust or pierce).
39. The Phoenix Spreads His Wings	Chi (strike).
40. Halt—Left and Right with Step	Use Chieh (intercept and attack).
41. Shoot the Wild Goose	No technique, serves as preparation and collection of energy.
42. The White Monkey Offers Fruit	Repetition—see position number 38.
43. Scatter Flowers—Left and Right	The technique Chi (strike) is contained in each of the movements performed from right to left and from left to right; Chi is used here against the inner side of the opponent's wrist or upper arm when the opponent wants to use a strike against your feet or legs.
44. Fair Lady Threads the Shuttle	By first circling the arms, the collection of energy is supported and then continues downward into Tz'u (thrust or pierce).

45. The White Tiger Hits with His Tail	First use Chi (strike) at the opponent's legs with the forward movement of the sword; when a new attack comes from the opponent, employ Ke (block); another technique is usually used immediately afterward.
46. The Tiger Puts His Head Between His Paws	Repetition—see position number 22.
47. The Carp Jumps Through the Dragon Gate	The same techniques are used as in position number 8.
48. The Black Dragon Twines Around a Column	First use Pi (split) to the back-left downward, then Pi from down to up, then Pi to the back-right downward, and toward the end use Tz'u (thrust or pierce) to the forward front. Variation: instead of Pi, use Hsi (clear and resolve), then T'i (lift), and then Tz'u (thrust or pierce).
49. The Holy Man Points Out the Way	Contains no technique.
50. The Wind Sweeps Away the Plum Blossoms	When several opponents are around you, use Chi (strike), moving in a circle.
51. The Tiger Puts His Head Between His Paws	Repetition—see position number 22.
52. Step Forward—the Compass Needle Points South	Use Tz'u (thrust or pierce).
53. Turn the Sword Over and Return to the Beginning Position	Contains no technique.

Remarks about Sword Fighting

1. **"The attack doesn't come from oneself"**: In accordance with the principles of T'ai Chi Ch'uan, you first move after the opponent moves. It is elementary that the initiative to fight doesn't come from oneself. This shows that the T'ai Chi sword is a true method of self-defense.

2. **Yielding, Following:** The principles of yielding and following have a central importance in the application of the techniques. It makes a distinctive approach toward the opponent possible and has a great deal to do with the way that T'ai Chi Ch'uan is thought of as a "friendly" sword art. This is also supported by the fact that the majority of the techniques are aimed at the arms and the legs.

3. **Balance:** Maintaining balance is of great importance in sword fighting. As in Push Hands (Tui Shou),[30] you try to bring your opponent off-balance, while maintaining your own equilibrium.

4. **"Before you go left, you should turn to the right (and vice versa)"**: This principle is important in the application and combination of the techniques.

5. **About the sword finger:** In the application of a technique, the sword finger, when the position permits it, is placed with emphasis on the hand, wrist, or lower-right arm holding the sword. This intensifies the directed movement of the energy. To strengthen the blocking of the position, for example, "The Rhinoceros Looks at the Moon," the sword finger is placed on the wrist.

6. **The position of the sword finger:** The various positions of the sword finger help to maintain and stabilize one's balance. Therefore, the arm (sword finger) is held backward during large sweeping movements with the sword, as in "The Phoenix Spreads Its Wings." Holding the sword finger near the right wrist, as is indicated in many positions, also serves to protect the sword finger, that is, the left hand, from the attacking sword.

7. **Clear and resolve:** In clear and resolve (Hsi), or during sword exercises with a partner, the blade of your own sword can briefly touch the opponent's sword although no pressure should be placed upon it nor should striking occur.

---

[30] See the glossary on pages 171–74.

8. Pa Kua sword forms: The techniques contained in the position "The Sword Circles Like a Cartwheel—Left and Right," are especially used against the Pa Kua sword forms.[31]

9. Japanese sword forms: Against the Japanese sword forms, the techniques in positions 4, 5, 8, and 13 can be particularly effective.

10. Speed: Practicing the sword form at the usual T'ai Chi speed serves to develop the ch'i. When using the techniques, one's speed is obviously adjusted to that of the opponent.

11. The sword and the body: The sword and the body form a unit during all the movements.

12. Reactions to attacks:
- Avoid an attack aimed at your head by bending your knees, stepping aside, and directing your own sword from below at your opponent's wrist or legs.
- Avoid an attack to the center of your body by taking a step to the side and trying, as well as possible, to get far behind your opponent.
- Avoid an attack aimed at your legs by getting out of the way and directing your sword at your opponent's wrist.
- Avoid an attack from above or the side by advancing rapidly toward the opponent with Chieh (halt and attack).

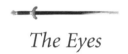

The Eyes

It is important that one's eyes be integrated into the movement.

Toward the end of the positions, you normally look at that part of the blade that is "active" in the technique used. For example, in Tz'u (thrust), you would look at the point of the sword and in Ke (block), at the lower part of the blade.

At the same time, the eyes shouldn't be locked into a stare. In a fighting situation, the practitioner must be able to react immediately when the situation changes.

When the sword isn't in the field of vision, as in the beginning of the sword form, you look straight forward at the horizon.

In general, there are two things you should try to keep in mind: be aware of the overall situation and, at the same time, accompany the performance of the movements with attentive watching, as indicated.

---

[31] "Pa Kua" belongs to the internal martial arts, with its sequence of movements performed mostly in a circle; see the glossary on pages 171–74.

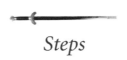

Steps

The steps Parallel Stance, Bow Step, T-Step, and Step of the Fishing Horse in the sword form are the same as those used in the short and long forms.

The Bow Step in the sword form varies according to the size of the steps. In the position "Looking for the Snake in the Grass," the steps have no special names but are considered a variation of the Bow Step.

Perhaps the term Bow Step (also called the forward stance) needs an additional explanation: it is the movement of energy within the legs, passing the lower tan t'ien area in a slight arc, which gives the Bow Step its name.

We can also think of the bending and stretching of the legs as similar to a bow preparing to shoot an arrow.

Horses standing in shallow water have the habit of repeatedly lifting one front leg out of the water and putting it down again. It seems as if they are fishing. In the Step of the Fishing Horse you have the weight of your body on your back leg, and your front leg is lifted so that only the front part of the foot touches the ground.

See foot diagram on page 49.

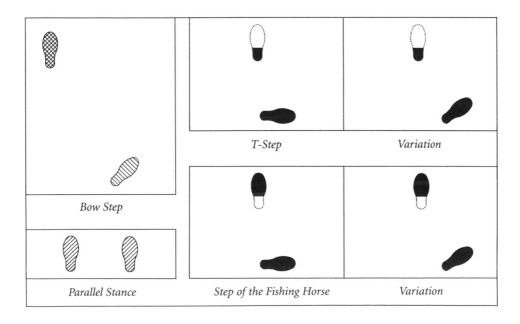

| T-Step | Variation |
| Bow Step | Step of the Fishing Horse | Variation |
| Parallel Stance |

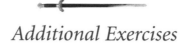

Additional Exercises

Practitioners who don't otherwise practice T'ai Chi Ch'uan can benefit from the following exercises. The order is optional.

1. Standing in the Parallel Stance: The knees are slightly bent, the lower back is relaxed, the arms hang down; release the groin fold. The groin fold is the crease that appears when you relax in the area between the upper thigh and the torso.
Stand 1 to 10 minutes, as long as possible: standing still can be interrupted by a short period of pacing back and forth; over months (or years), work up to 20 minutes of standing.

2. Standing on one leg: Lift your thigh so that it is parallel to the floor or somewhat higher; the calf and foot hang down; your arms hang beside your body. Stand this way for 1 to 2 minutes, and then change sides.

3. Standing in the T-Step: Ninety percent of your body weight rests on your back foot, 10 percent (or the actual weight of your front leg) is on the front foot; the heel touches the floor; the arms hang relaxed next to the body. Ninety percent of your body weight rests on your back foot; 10 percent (or the actual weight of your front leg) rests on the front foot. The heel touches the floor; the arms hang relaxed next to the body. Hold this position for 1 to 2 minutes (see "Circling the Moon Three Times").

4. Crouching: In a wide bow step, crouch down several times, keeping most of your weight on your back leg. Practice this on the left and right (see "The Swallow Takes Water").

5. Eye Exercises: Eye exercises were already suggested for sword fighters in ancient China. It is best to practice them while seated.

1. With closed eyes, let the eyeballs circle seven times to the left and then to the right.
2. Open your eyes and focus upon an object in the distance, and then one very close; do this several times.
3. Blink rapidly, looking as far left as possible and then as far right as possible, while holding your head still; repeat this several times.

6. An exercise for stability when performing the steps: Practice walking by first placing the outer edges of your feet on the floor. This way of walking, which is felt to be rather unusual at first, is an old secret for increasing the stability and agility of your steps. It has been handed down from General Li.

Partner Exercises with the Sword

1. Both partners stand opposite each other and bring their swords together at the middle of the blades. Beginners can tie their swords together with a string.

2. The partners walk through the room together. With a slight pressure and turning movement of the blade, also combined with lifting and sinking, one partner "attacks;" the opponent reacts, without losing contact with the partner's sword (the swords should stick together). This exercise trains one in the feeling and sticking energy; it makes the importance of the sword's safeguard clear, which is to catch the attacks of the opponent's sword. It is advisable for beginners to decide who will take the initiative and who will follow the movement of the other. This was one of Cheng Man-Ch'ing's favorite sword exercises.

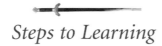

Steps to Learning

1. Learn the sword form correctly.
2. Learn the 13 techniques contained in the positions.
3. Pay special attention to the quality of each technique while practicing alone.
4. Working with a partner, study the various applications and combination possibilities of the positions and the techniques. Some teachers have put together a little "exercise series" that is similar to the San T'sai Sword.[32]
5. With a partner, practice the free application of the positions, that is, the techniques, while taking the principles into consideration.

An improvement in the T'ai Chi sword form can't be accomplished by the completion of these steps alone. When you don't otherwise practice T'ai Chi, it will require daily exercising (repetition) of the sword form over the years.

Difficulties Faced by Beginners in Practicing the Sword

- The sword is held tensely (in a clench).
- There is uncertainty about the correct "play" of the handle in the hand.
- The coordination of sword and body movement is difficult.
- Even arcs can't be formed with the sword or the tip of the sword.

---

[32] See the glossary on pages 171–74.

These difficulties disappear with increased practice: The sword is ever more clearly experienced as a part of the body. It lies lightly in the hand. Its circular arcing movement comes naturally from the movement of the body.

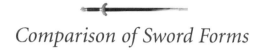

Comparison of Sword Forms

The sword form of Dr. Chi, as described here, shows a sequence identical to that written down by Chen Wei-Ming. The external form of the positions is the same. The names of the positions in this book are commonly used in the T'ai Chi sword. They agree with the positions named by Chen Wei-Ming.

Dr. Chi's sword form agrees basically with the one shown by Cheng Man-Ch'ing. Both of them convey the same form and sequence of positions. The differences are in the points of the compass to which individual positions are directed and in the forming of the transitions. Cheng Man-Ch'ing first transfers the weight in the transitions entirely backward, emphasizing the principle of yielding, as in his short form. The transitions in Cheng Man-Ch'ing show correspondingly larger movements with the sword.

Also, in the sword form of Fu Zhong-Wen, who was a senior student of Yang Cheng-Fu (as was Cheng Man-Ch'ing), the same positions and the same sequence are used as in Dr. Chi's form, except for two differences.[33] Some transitions in Fu Zhong-Wen contain additional movements with the sword. Fu also directs individual positions with an accentuated movement of the wrist using the technique Chi (strike). Above all, in the second half of his form he varies some of the directions of the compass in which the positions are performed.

This comparison, which could be continued in this fashion with other well-known sword masters, makes it clear that the positions contained in this book are fundamental for the classical T'ai Chi sword, and the sequence can be seen as its basic structure. The transitions between the positions shown by Dr. Chi are similar to those of master T. T. Liang[34] and are confined to leading into the next position. They are relatively easily shaped, which suits their presentation in book form.

[33] He performs "Shake Off the Dust in the Wind" differently, and instead of "Looking for the Snake in the Grass" he uses the position "Dragon Walk."
[34] See the glossary on pages 171–74.

List of the Positions in the Sword Form

1. Awaken the Ch'i at the Beginning
2. Circling the Moon Three Times
3. Great Star of the Big Dipper
4. The Swallow Takes Water
5. Detain and Come Forward—Left and Right
6. Small Star of the Big Dipper
7. The Swallow Flies into the Nest
8. The Clever Cat Catches a Mouse
9. The Dragonfly Touches the Water
10. The Bee Flies into the Hive
11. The Phoenix Spreads Its Wings
12. Whirlwind Left
13. Small Star of the Big Dipper
14. Whirlwind Right
15. Waiting for the Fish
16. Looking for the Snake in the Grass
17. Embrace the Moon
18. The Bird Flies into the Forest to Rest
19. The Black Dragon Hits with His Tail
20. The Wind Moves the Lotus
21. The Lion Shakes His Mane
22. The Tiger Puts His Head Between His Paws
23. The Wild Horse Springs over the Mountain Stream
24. Turn Around and Rein In the Horse
25. Step Forward—the Compass Needle Points South
26. Shake Off the Dust in the Wind
27. Send the Boat Downstream
28. The Shooting Star Follows the Moon
29. The Heavenly Horse Flies Through the Air
30. Move the Curtain
31. The Sword Circles Like a Cartwheel—Left and Right
32. The Mythical Bird Spreads One Wing
33. Lifting the Moon from the Bottom of the Sea
34. Embrace the Moon
35. The Demon Looks into the Water
36. The Rhinoceros Looks at the Moon
37. Shoot the Swallow
38. The White Monkey Offers Fruit
39. The Phoenix Spreads Its Wings
40. Halt—Left and Right with Step
41. Shoot the Wild Goose
42. The White Monkey Offers Fruit
43. Scatter Flowers—Left and Right
44. Fair Lady Threads the Shuttle
45. The White Tiger Hits with His Tail
46. The Tiger Puts His Head Between His Paws
47. The Carp Jumps Through the Dragon Gate
48. The Black Dragon Twines Around a Column
49. The Holy Man Points Out the Way

The positions of the sword form pictured here, like all positions in classical T'ai Chi, show a special relationship of the limbs of the body to each other. This reminds us of the golden mean (happy medium). The golden mean represents an especially harmonious relationship of various parts to each other. That T'ai Chi forms are found to be harmonious and aesthetically pleasing to the observer is due, among other things, to this.

The Presentation of the Sword Form

According to the principles of T'ai Chi Ch'uan, the movement is directed by the center of the body (hip area—lower tan t'ien). The torso moves with it as one unit. The movements of the arms, sword, and legs follow the movement of the torso. Only the "empty leg" and the "empty arm" move independently.

Each of the separate movements described under each photograph begins and ends at the same time.

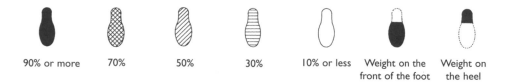

| 90% or more | 70% | 50% | 30% | 10% or less | Weight on the front of the foot | Weight on the heel |

The foot diagram under the photographs shows the appropriate distribution of weight and the position of the feet, at that particular point.

The hip diagram (shaded area) is thought of as an additional aid, within the compass diagram, to make the sequence of the movements clearer. It shows the particular position of the torso. (Please note that this map refers to the photographs.)

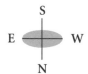

The sword diagram presents the position of the sword when it can't be clearly recognized in the photograph.

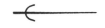

The arrows show the direction of the sequence of movement leading into the next photograph.

To help in understanding the orientation, we use the points of the compass. Independently of the actual points of the compass, the direction in which one begins the exercise is called north.

In some of the photographs, due to the angle of the photograph, the feet, torso, arms, or sword might be difficult to recognize. In case of doubt, what counts are the descriptions and the diagrams.

In addition to its practical aspect as a learning aid,
the demonstration of the sword form through pictures
has an additional significance. It retains for us
what normally exists only in movement.
It gives us information about the construction of
the sword form and the shape of the positions.
Since the positions shown here are basic for the T'ai Chi
sword, showing them in a book helps our orientation.
It makes it possible to compare sword forms and
allows us to reach conclusions about the
modifications that have taken place.

1. AWAKEN THE CH'I AT THE BEGINNING

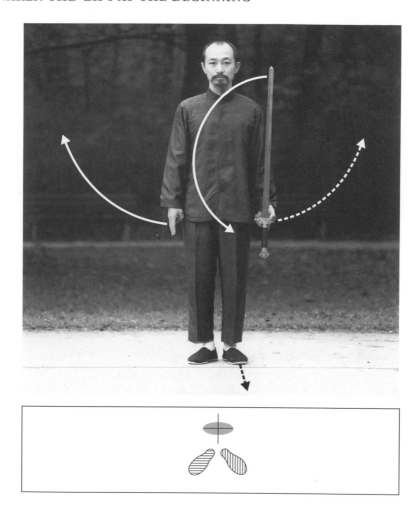

1. The heels are together. The knees are slightly bent. The lower back is relaxed. The spine is held straight. The weight is evenly distributed on both feet. The blade of the sword is held perpendicular to the ground.* The right hand forms the sword finger.**

---

* Although one usually practices with a dull metal sword or a wooden sword, one conducts oneself as if the blade were sharp. The cutting edge shouldn't touch the body. See the "Holding the Sword" section for how to hold the sword in the beginning.

** See "The Sword Finger" section for information about the sword finger.

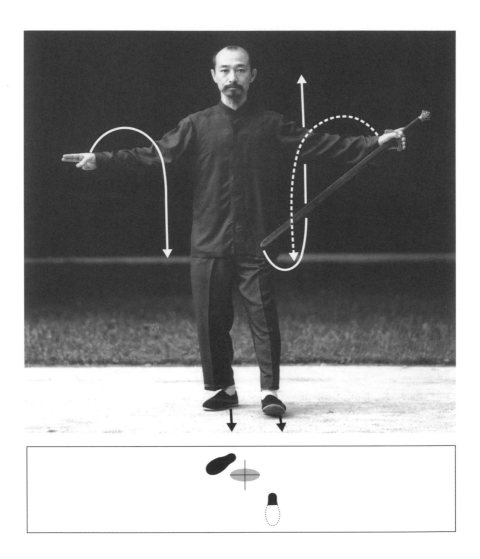

2. Shift your weight onto your right foot and place your left leg forward with the left heel first. Lift both arms to the NW and NE and bend them somewhat at the same time. First, bring the sword blade slightly forward, and then lower it to the right, in front of your body.

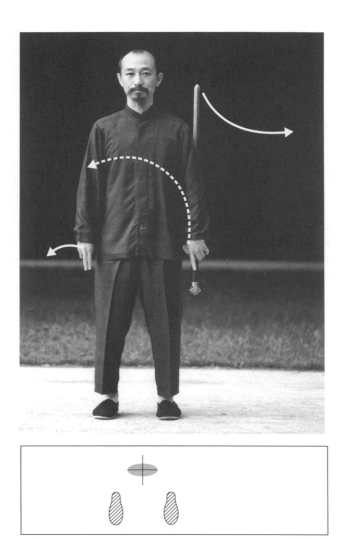

3. Shift your weight onto your left foot and place your right foot parallel to your left foot. While doing this, draw an inward circular arc with both arms, directing the movement from the elbows. Along with this, lower your arms. Guide the sword behind your left arm. (The blade touches the upper part of the lower arm and the elbow.)

You are in the position "Awaken the Ch'i at the Beginning."

Note: The transitions that lead from one position into the next are counted as part of the position. Some positions contain variations or repetitions performed to the right and left.

2. Circling the Moon Three Times

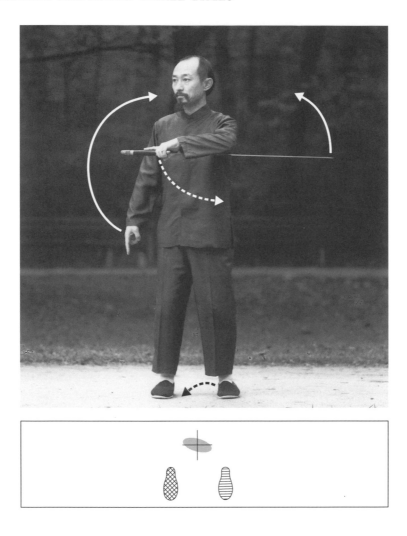

1. Turn your torso slightly to the right; at the same time, shift your weight onto your right foot. Lift your right arm somewhat and turn it clockwise. Lift your left arm with the sword and move it to the right; at the same time, bend the arm at the elbow.

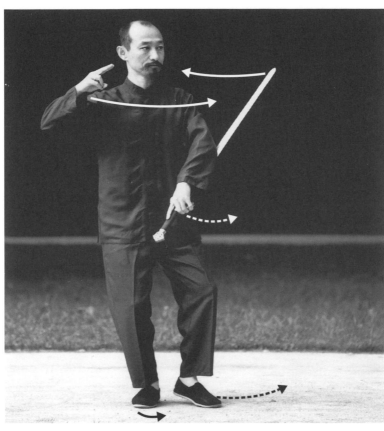

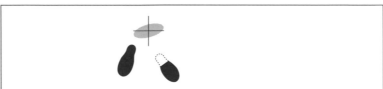

2. Shift your weight further onto your right foot. Turn your torso left; while doing this, pivot on the front part of your left foot.* Lift your right arm NE and, by bending it (release the elbow), guide the hand to your head. Lower your left arm with the sword.

* The front part of the foot includes the ball of the foot and the toes lying flat on the floor.

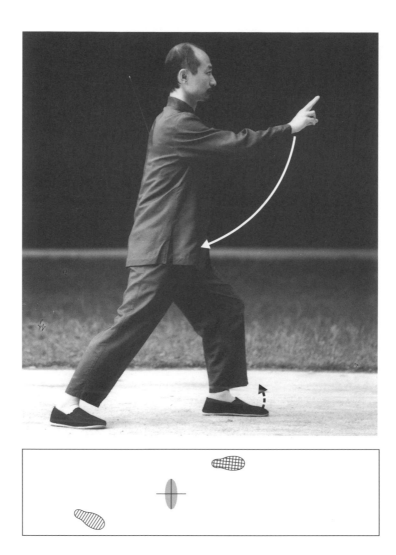

3. Place your left leg to the W with the heel first. Shift up to 70 percent of your weight onto your left foot, and pivot your right foot on the heel until the toes point NW (bow step). While doing this, turn your torso left and bring your right arm forward to the W. Along with shifting your weight and turning your torso, guide the sword to the left side of your body.

Note: The sequence of this movement is similar to the "brush knee" in the short and long forms.

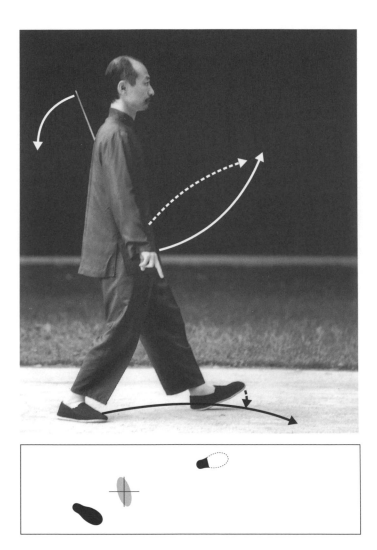

4. Shift up to 90 percent of your weight onto your right foot; while doing this, lower your right arm. Toward the end of the movement, lift the front part of your left foot; turn your torso somewhat to the left and point your toes SW.

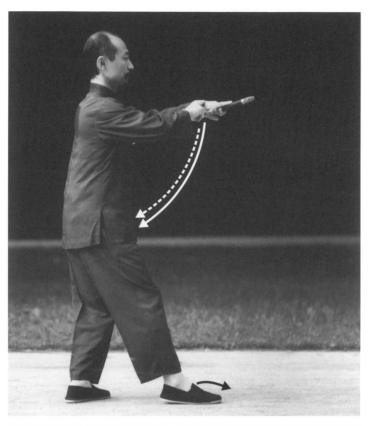

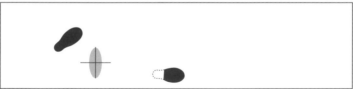

5. Shift your weight onto your left foot and place your right leg in front W, on the front part of your foot (Step of the Fishing Horse). At the same time, lift both arms, slightly rounded, to somewhat below shoulder height (relax your shoulders). The blade of the sword continues to lie on the lower arm as described. The sword finger touches the lower-right part of the back of the left hand with the upper part of the forefinger and the middle finger (see sketch).

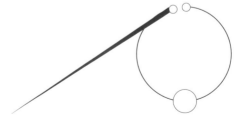

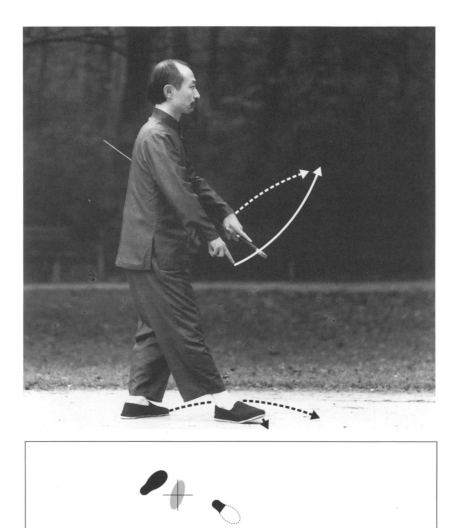

6. Turn your torso a little to the right and lower your arms with the sword. Separate your arms.

Simultaneously lift your right leg and place it forward to the right, heel first.

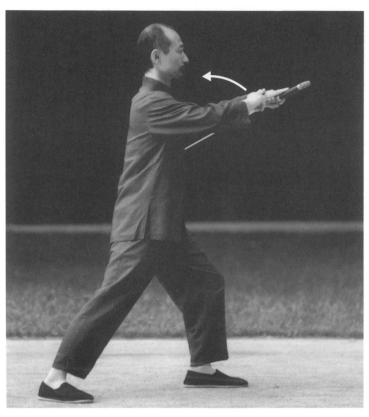

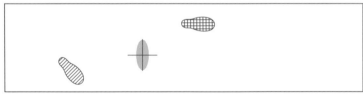

7. (a) Shift your weight onto your right foot and place your left leg forward to the W, heel first (Bow Step).

(b) Without pausing, shift your weight onto your left foot. While doing this, lift both arms, somewhat rounded, to just under shoulder height, over the outside.

Note: The difference between this illustration and illustration 5 is that the blade of the sword is held away from the lower part of the arm (see sketch). The position of the sword finger is the same as in illustration 5.

You are in the position "Circling the Moon Three Times."

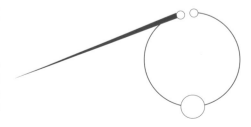

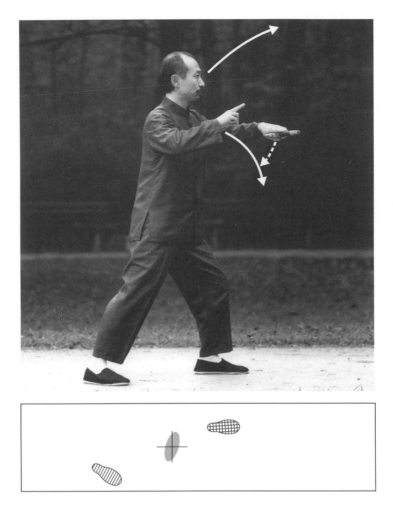

1. Turn your torso somewhat to the right. Lower both arms slightly and remove the sword finger from the back of your left hand by releasing your elbow.

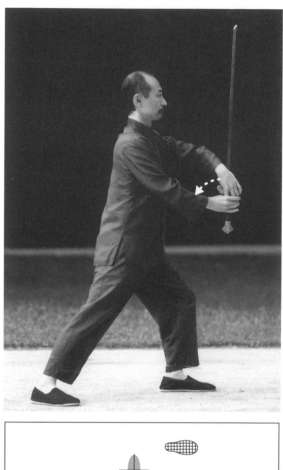

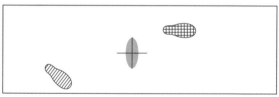

2. Turn your torso to the front again. Along with this, grasp the sword handle with your right hand over your left forefinger. With your left hand, bring the sword into a perpendicular position. Simultaneously pass it into your right hand and release it.

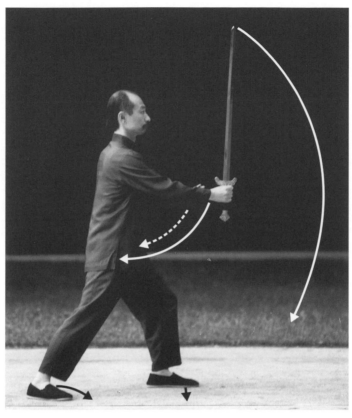

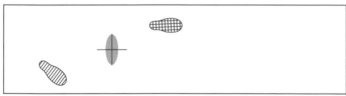

3. Remove your left hand forming the sword finger and direct it at your right wrist.

Note: Illustrations 1–3 show a relatively rapid series of movements.

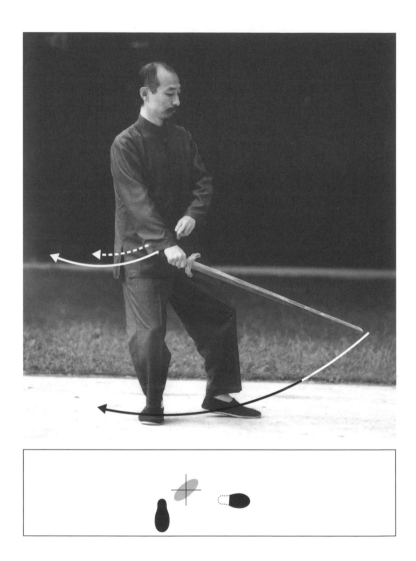

4. (a) Shift your weight completely onto your left foot. At the same time, turn your torso to the right, lift your right leg, and place it forward, heel first, with the toes pointing N.

(b) Shift your weight onto your right foot; at the same time, turn your torso further to the right and place your left leg forward to the right on the front part of your left foot. (Step of the Fishing Horse.) Simultaneously lower the sword in a forward arc.

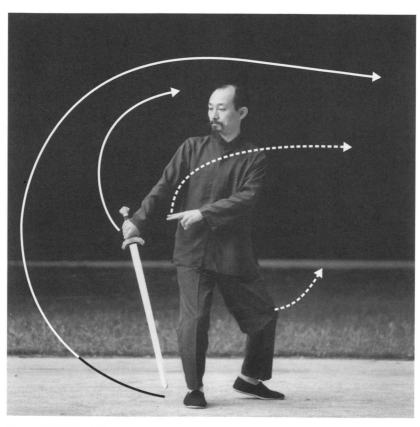

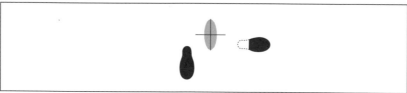

5. Turn your torso further to the right. Your arms and the sword follow the movement of your torso.

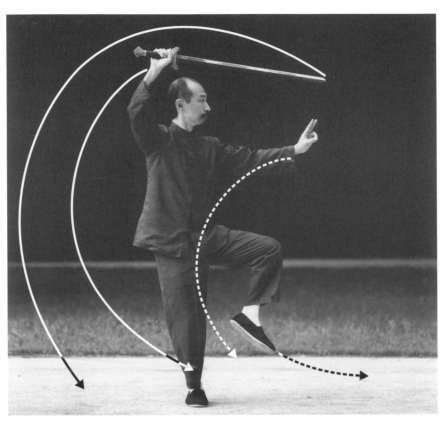

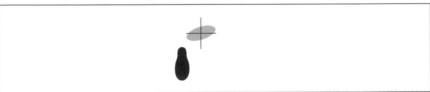

6. (a) Shift your weight further onto your right foot. Turn the sword clockwise until the back of your hand faces S.

(b) Shift the weight completely onto the right foot. Through a slight stretching of the right leg, lift the left leg and direct the sword with a standing blade* from the back E forward W. While doing this, turn your torso to the left. Along with this, remove the sword finger from your right wrist, bring it forward and point it at the tip of the sword.

You are in the position "Great Star of the Big Dipper."

Note: When you guide the sword to the front, do it next to your body and not over your head.

---

* The terms standing and lying for blade position help the practitioner to find the correct orientation for his or her sword. Lying and standing blades refer to different angles and heights, as can be seen in the photographs. If you put a sword or knife down on a flat surface, the blade "lies" flat on its side; if you cut into an object vertically from top to bottom, the blade "stands."

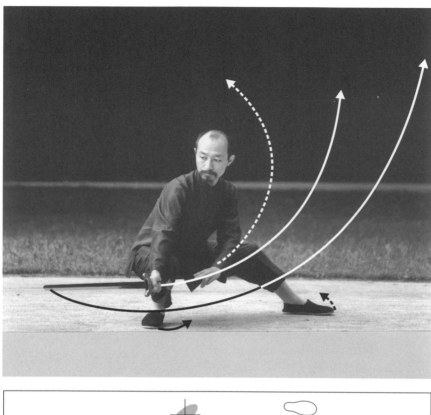

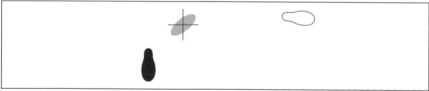

1. Crouch down and place your left foot to the W, your toes facing WNW. Lower the sword toward the NNE (stretch your arm only near the end of the movement; otherwise the arc becomes too large). By releasing your left elbow, direct the sword finger at your right wrist again.

Note: It is not necessary to go as low in the crouch as is shown in the photograph.

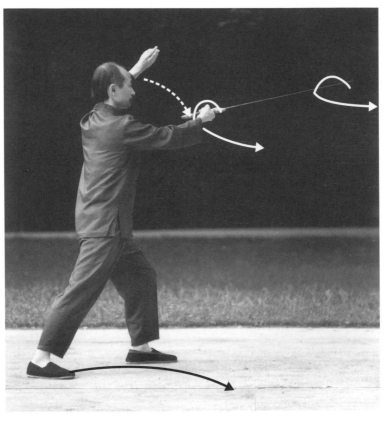

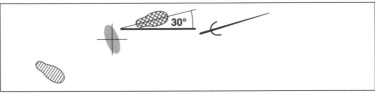

2. Shift your weight onto your left foot and at the same time, turn it outward on the heel SW (30°*). Simultaneously, turn your torso left and, coming up from the crouch, turn your right foot on its heel. While you shift your weight and turn your torso, direct the sword first near the floor (the swallow takes water) and then diagonally up to the front left. The rounded left arm follows the movement of your torso, and you lift the sword finger above your head to the left.

You are in the position "The Swallow Takes Water."

---

* As you can see in the section "Steps," the position of the feet is directed either to the main compass points (N, S, E, W) or to the points between (NE, NW, SW, SE), also called 45° or diagonal. A number of positions differ slightly from this rule. On certain techniques, one foot or both feet can be in the position 30°, see the foot diagram on this page. This would be either 30° to the left or to the right of the closest main compass point from the previous foot position.

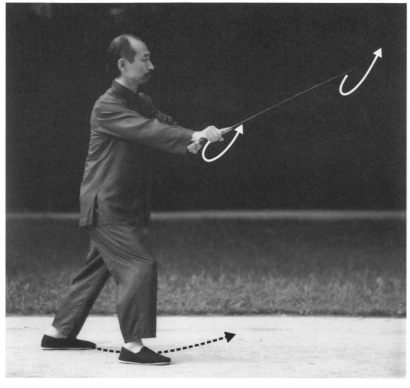

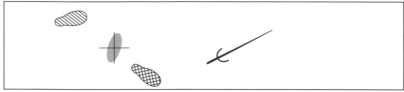

1. (a) Shift your weight completely onto your left foot (releasing in the groin fold); at the same time, turn your torso a little to the left. Simultaneously, draw a small, counterclockwise arc with your right arm and the sword until the back of your hand faces up.

(b) Place your right leg forward, heel first (toes at 30°); turn your torso to the right and shift up to 70 percent of your weight onto your right foot. Direct the sword to the right; lower the sword finger level of your right wrist and point at it.

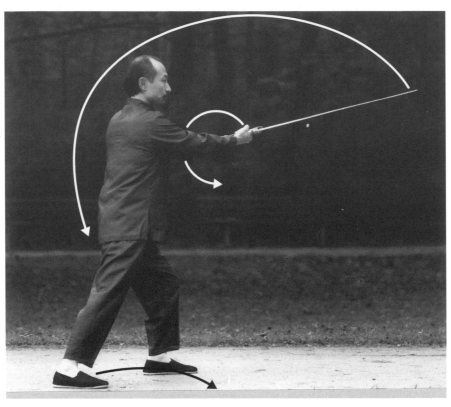

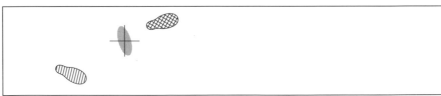

2. (a) Shift your weight completely onto the right foot, turning your torso a little to the right while doing this. Simultaneously, draw a small, clockwise arc with your right arm and the sword until the back of your hand faces down.

(b) Place your left leg forward, heel first (toes at 30°); turn your torso to the left and shift up to 70 percent of your weight onto your left foot. Direct the sword to the left. The sword finger remains pointed at your right wrist.

You are in the position "Detain and Come Forward—Left and Right."

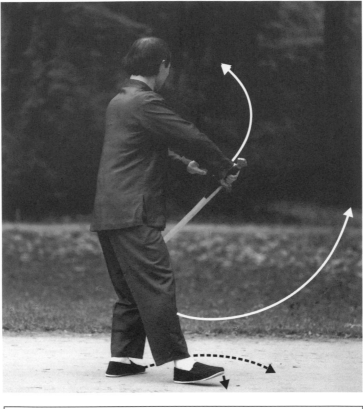

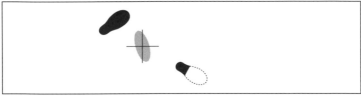

1. Shift your weight completely onto your left foot, turning your torso somewhat to the left and placing your right foot forward, heel first (toes pointing NW). Lower the sword, making an arc on the left side of your body. The sword finger remains pointed at your right wrist.

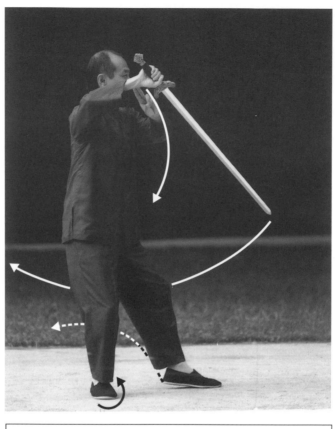

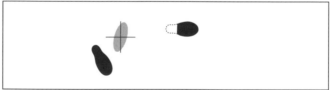

2. Shift your weight to your right foot, and place your left leg with the front part of your foot W (Step of the Fishing Horse). While doing this, turn your torso to the right. Lift your right arm, with the sword; the sword finger remains pointed at your wrist.

This is the position "Small Star of the Big Dipper."

Note: In a well-known variation of this position, the sword finger points at the tip of the sword, and the left leg is raised.

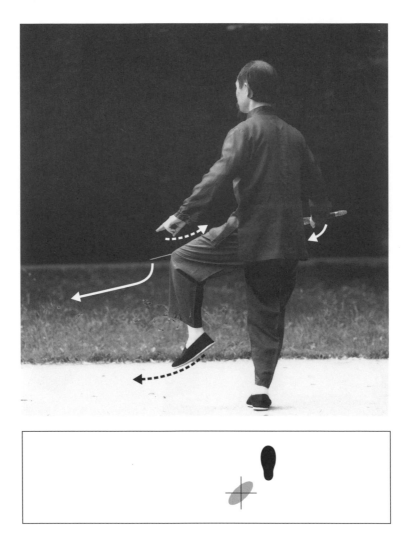

1. Turn your torso SE, thereby also turning your right foot on its heel until your toes point S. The left leg follows the movement and is raised at the same time. Simultaneously with turning your torso, lower both arms and move them apart. The sword remains on the right side of your body. Bring the blade into a lying position.

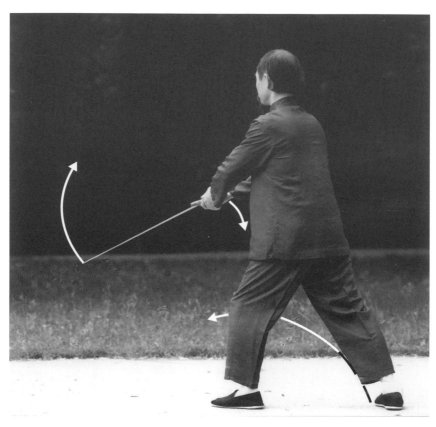

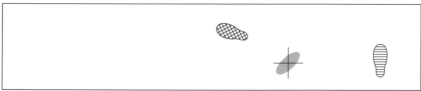

2. (a) Place your left leg forward, heel first, the toes pointing ESE.

(b) Shift your weight onto your left foot. Simultaneously, bring both arms together through small arcs from below upward. While doing this, turn the sword clockwise until the back of your hand faces down. Also open the sword finger and place the left hand under the right hand. While shifting your weight, direct the sword diagonally forward and downward.

You are in the position "The Swallow Flies into the Nest."

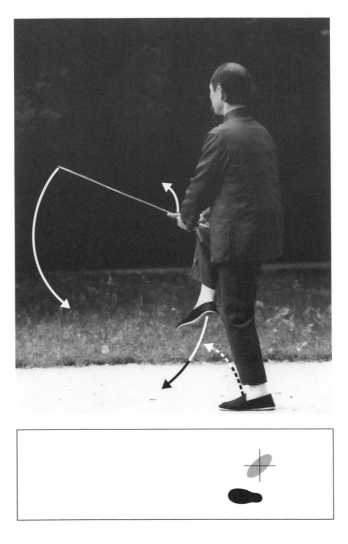

1. Shift your weight onto your left foot. Lift your right leg. While doing this, bring your arms somewhat closer to your body and lower them; simultaneously, raise the tip of the sword; the blade lies flat.

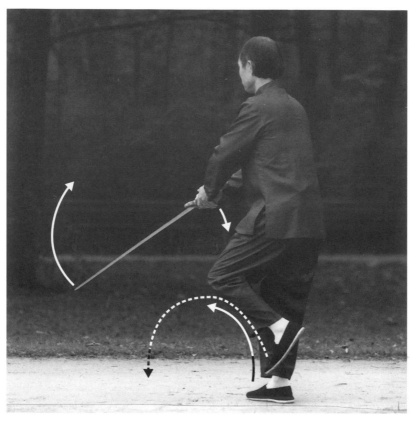

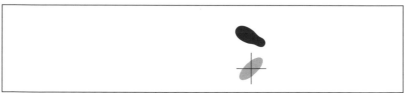

2. The following movement prepares you for the jump. First lower your right leg, shift your weight onto your right foot; while doing this, lower the blade of the sword, then pick up your left foot.

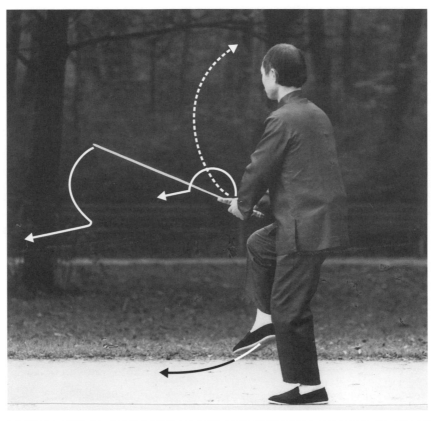

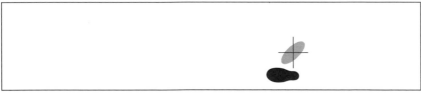

3. Spring from your right leg (foot) onto your left leg, again raising the blade at the same time.

Note: "The Clever Cat Catches a Mouse" contains a flat jump; "The Wild Horse Springs over the Mountain Stream," a wider and higher jump; and "The Carp Jumps Through the Dragon Gate," a high jump.

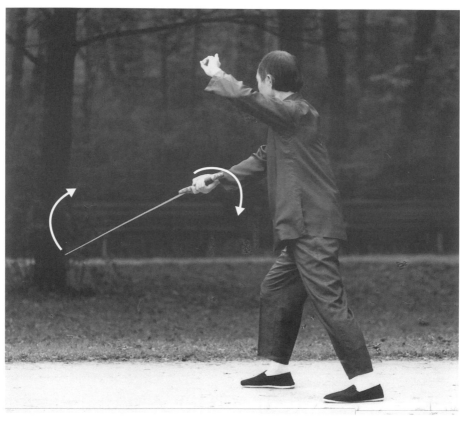

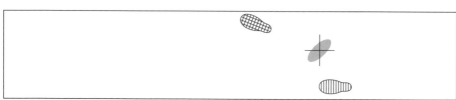

4. Slow down the movement and, from your left foot, place your right leg forward, heel first, toes pointing SE (Bow Step), and shift your weight. While doing this, direct the sword forward and downward so that the blade lies flat and the back of your right hand faces down. Release the left hand from the right hand, form the sword finger, and bring up the left arm.

You are in the position "The Clever Cat Catches a Mouse."

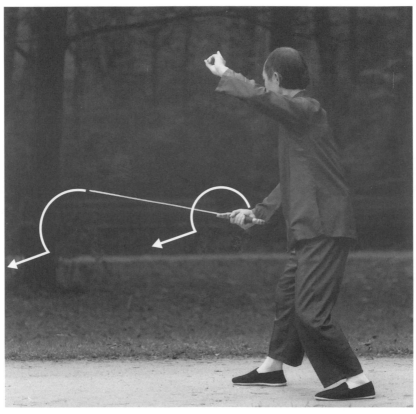

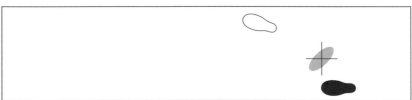

1. Shift your weight backward. Pull your arm and lower the handle of the sword to your body, raising the tip of the blade at the same time.

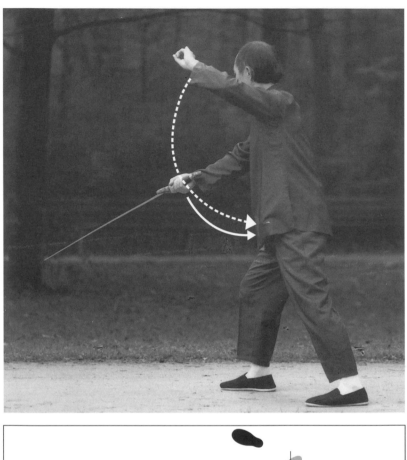

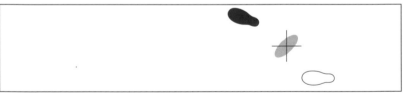

2. Shift your weight forward and, while doing this, direct the sword forward and downward. The blade lies flat.

You are in the position "The Dragonfly Touches the Water."

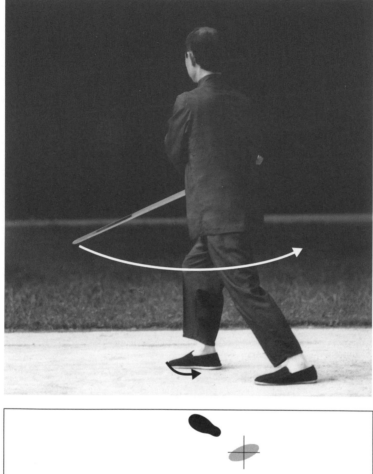

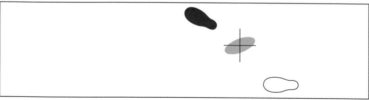

1. Turn your torso somewhat to the right, directing your right arm with the sword to the right side of your body. At the same time, turn the right hand and the sword counterclockwise until the back of the hand faces up. Lower your rounded left arm and point the sword finger at your right wrist.

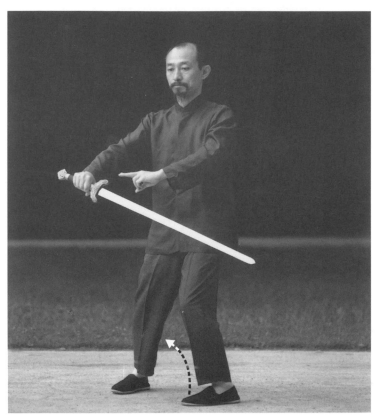

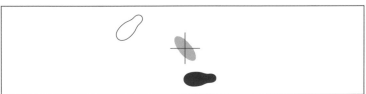

2. Shift your weight onto your left foot. Turn your torso left and turn on the heel of your right foot until your toes point NE. The arms and the sword follow the movement of the torso.*

* The difference between this position and "The Wind Sweeps Away the Plum Blossoms" is that here the blade is held diagonally. You only follow the opponent!

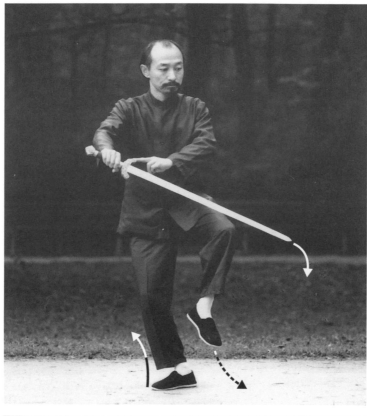

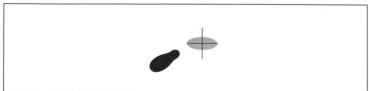

3. Shift your weight onto your right foot, turn your torso further to the left, and lift your left leg.

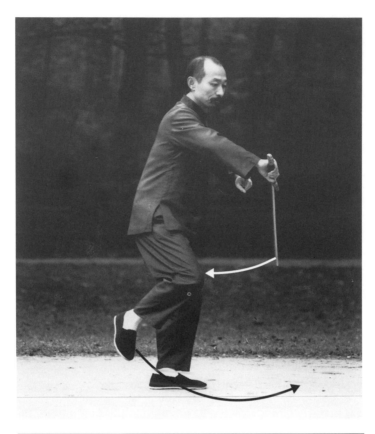

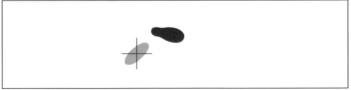

4. (a) Set down your left foot, heel first, in the same place, with the toes pointing WNW. Your arms and the sword follow the movement.

(b) Shift your weight to your left foot, turn your torso further to the left, and lift your right leg.

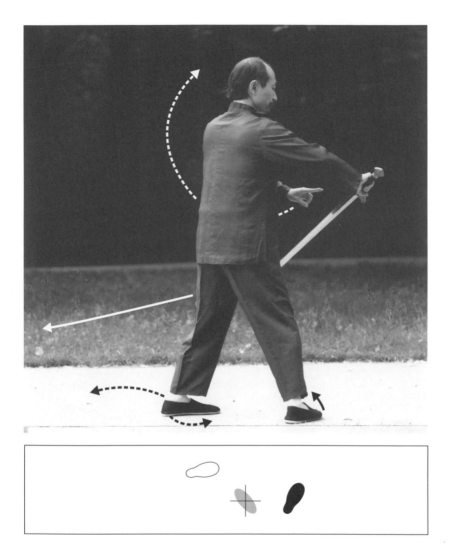

5. (a) Turn your torso further to the left. Place your right leg forward, moving it in an outward arc with the heel forward toward W with the toes pointing SSW. Your arms and the sword follow the movement of your torso.

(b) Shift your weight onto your right foot.

(Not shown): Shift your weight further onto your right foot, thereby turning your torso left; pivot on the front part of your left foot until your toes point SE (Step of the Fishing Horse).

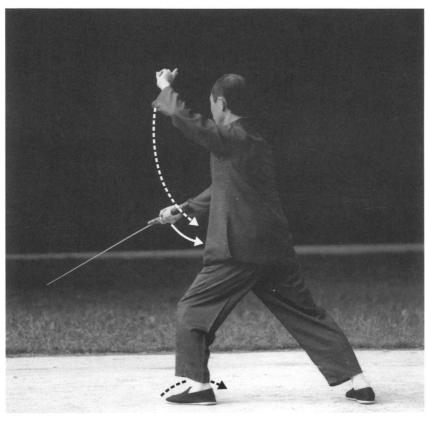

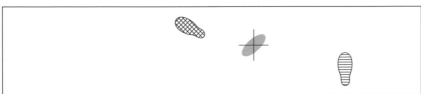

6. (a) Place your left leg so the heel faces SE.

(b) Shift your weight onto your left foot; the front part of the right foot turns slightly inward until the toes point S. Direct the sword forward and downward to the SE. While doing this, bend your right arm and turn the blade to a lying position by turning your right hand clockwise (the back of your hand faces down). Lift your rounded left arm (sword finger).

You are in the position "The Bee Flies into the Hive."

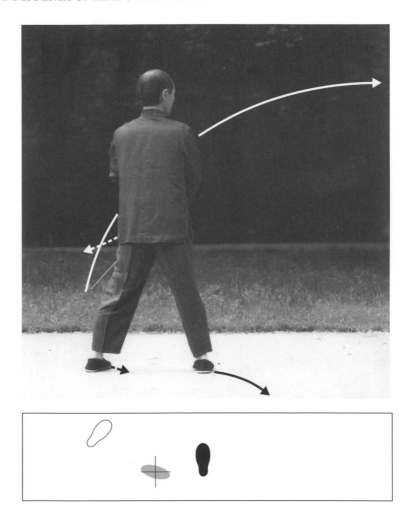

1. Shift your weight onto your right foot, turn your torso to the right, and pivot on the heel of your left foot, until your toes point SW. Simultaneously, lower your left arm and point the sword finger at your right wrist. The tip of the sword remains pointed to the SE.

(Not shown): Shift your weight onto your left foot, turn your torso further to the right, place your right leg, heel first, in an outward arc to the NW. Your arms and the sword remain on the left side of your body.

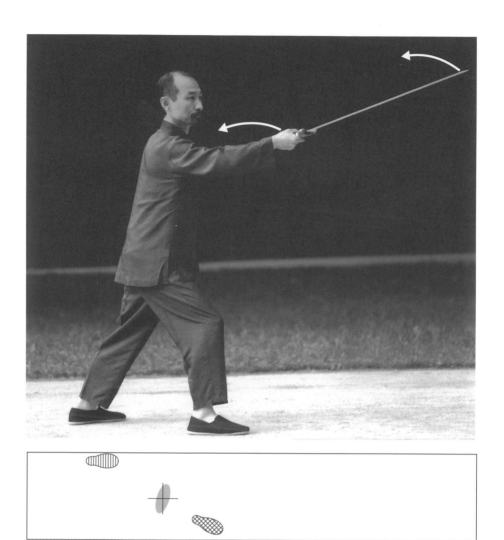

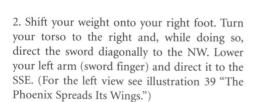

2. Shift your weight onto your right foot. Turn your torso to the right and, while doing so, direct the sword diagonally to the NW. Lower your left arm (sword finger) and direct it to the SSE. (For the left view see illustration 39 "The Phoenix Spreads Its Wings.")

You are in the position "The Phoenix Spreads Its Wings."

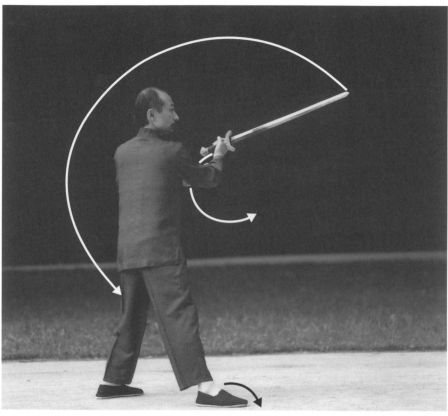

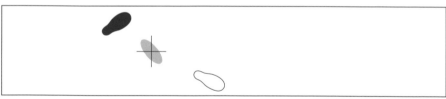

(Not shown): Shift your weight completely onto your right foot, lifting your left foot at the same time.

1. (a) Place your left foot SE, on the front part of your foot, with your toes pointing SW.

(b) Shift your weight onto your left foot and turn your torso left. While doing this, pull the sword to the left side of your body and bring the blade into a standing position. The sword finger remains pointed at your right wrist.

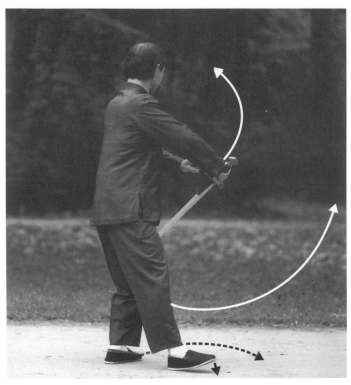

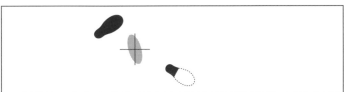

2. (a) Shift your weight completely onto your left foot, turn your torso further to the left and lift your right leg. At the same time, direct the sword further left and lower it.

(b) Turn your torso slightly right and set down your right leg with the heel in the same place, the toes pointing WNW. Direct the sword forward, continuing the arc from below, moving upward.

You are in the position "Whirlwind Left."

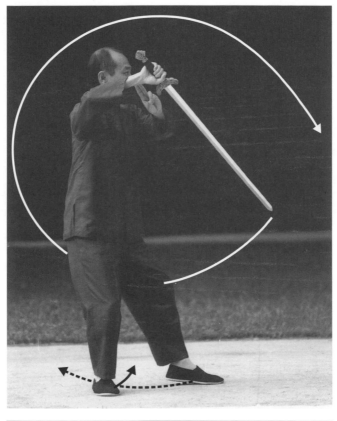

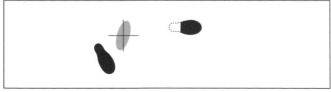

1. Shift your weight onto your right leg, turn your torso to the right, and place your left leg forward (Step of the Fishing Horse). At the same time, direct the sword forward and upward.

You are in the position "Small Star of the Big Dipper."

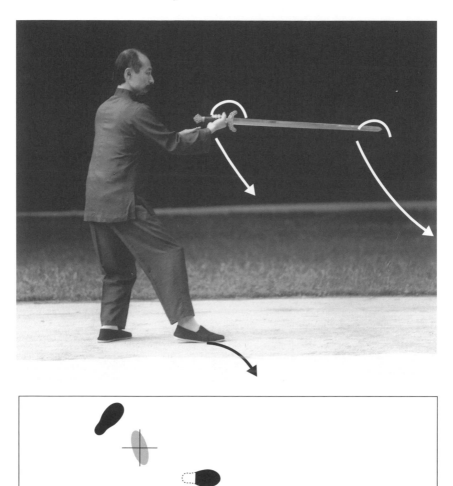

1. (a) Turn your torso left and place your left leg back to the SE, with the front part of the foot first. Your toes point SW. At the same time, lower your arms and direct the sword to the left side of your body. Shift your weight to your left foot, without a pause, turn your torso further left, and direct the sword backward. The sword finger remains pointed at your right wrist.

(b) Turn your torso to the right; while doing this, place your right leg left, with the front part of the foot first. (Step of the Fishing Horse). While turning your torso, direct the sword in an arc upward and forward (the blade stands). The sword finger remains pointed at your right wrist.

You are in the position "Whirlwind Right."

2. From this position, you move without hesitation directly into the position "Waiting for the Fish."

Note: Directing the sword in a circular arc on the left side of your body is "Whirlwind Right." The last part of the movement is the position "Waiting for the Fish."

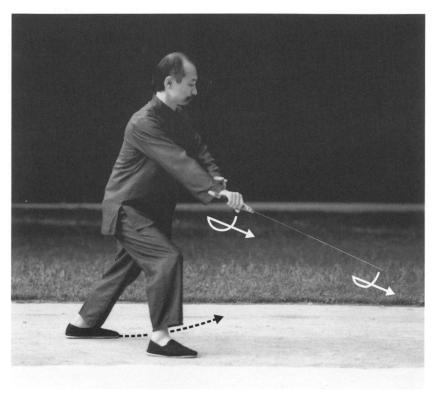

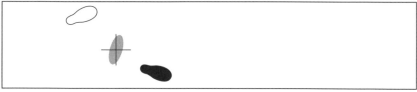

1. Move your right leg forward to the right, heel first, toes 30°. Shift your weight onto your right foot, turn your torso to the right, and direct the sword forward and downward. The sword finger remains pointed at your right wrist.

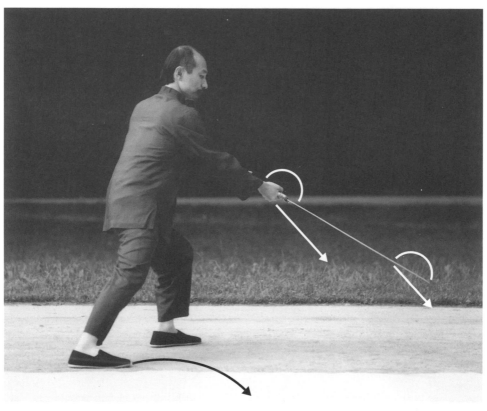

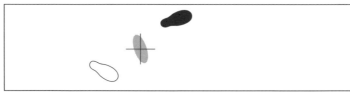

(Not shown): Shift your weight further onto your right foot; turn your torso slightly to the right (release in the groin fold). Simultaneously pull your arms and the sword somewhat toward your body by bending your elbows; raise the tip of the sword a bit while doing so, then draw a small clockwise arc with the sword until the back of your hand faces down.

2. Place your left leg forward to the left, heel first (toes 30°). Shift your weight onto your left foot. Turn your torso left and, while turning, direct the sword downward. The sword finger continues to point at your wrist.

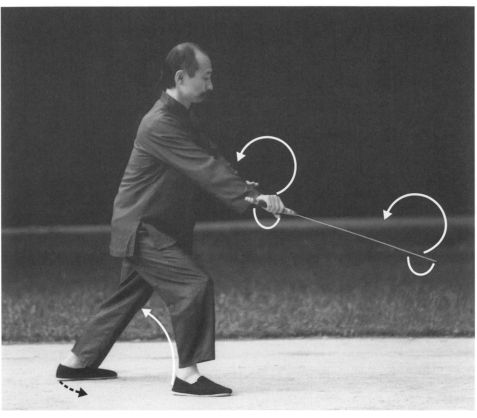

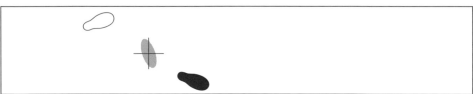

(Not shown): Shift your weight further onto your left foot and turn your torso somewhat to the left (release in the groin fold). Simultaneously pull your arms and the sword somewhat closer to your body by bending your elbows; while doing so raise the tip of the sword a bit; then, draw a small counterclockwise arc with the sword until the back of your hand faces up.

3. Place your right leg forward, heel first, (toes 30°). Repeat; see illustration 1.

You are in the position "Looking for the Snake in the Grass."

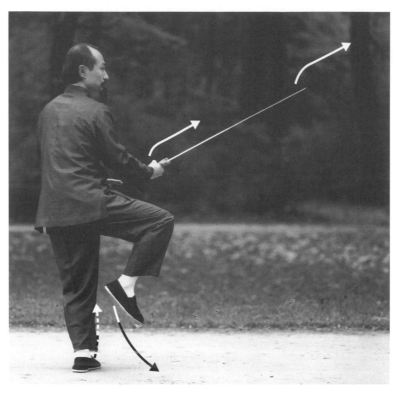

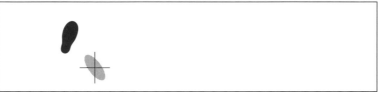

1. (a) First turn the heel of your left foot W until the toes point SSW.

(b) Shift your weight onto your left foot; at the same time turn your torso to the left and draw up your right leg. Simultaneously, turn your arm and the sword clockwise; then direct them in a convex arc to the left side of your body. While doing this, raise the tip of the sword (the blade lies flat).

You are in the position "Embrace the Moon."

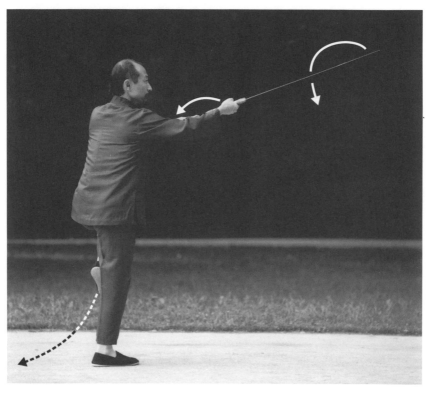

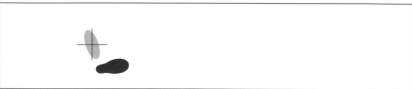

1. (a) Place your right leg forward to the W, heel first (toes somewhat inward).

(b) Shift your weight onto your right leg and turn your torso somewhat right. At the same time, stretch the right leg slightly and draw up the left leg (the knee faces SW). Simultaneously, direct the sword upward. The sword finger remains pointed at your wrist.

You are in the position "The Bird Flies into the Forest to Rest."

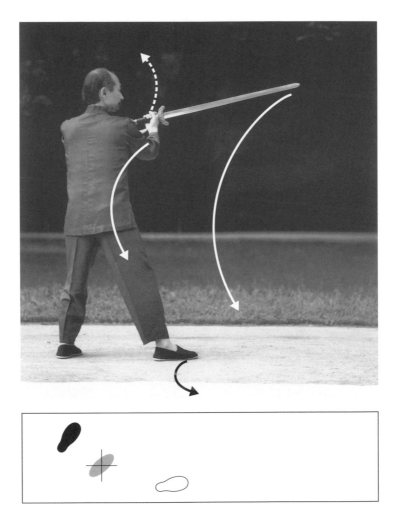

1. (a) Bend your right leg and place your left leg left backward, with the front part of the foot first (toes point SW).

(b) Shift your weight onto your left foot. Turn your torso left, lower your arms and the sword, and pull them to the left side of your body; bring the blade of the sword into a vertical position at the same time. The sword finger remains pointed at your right wrist.

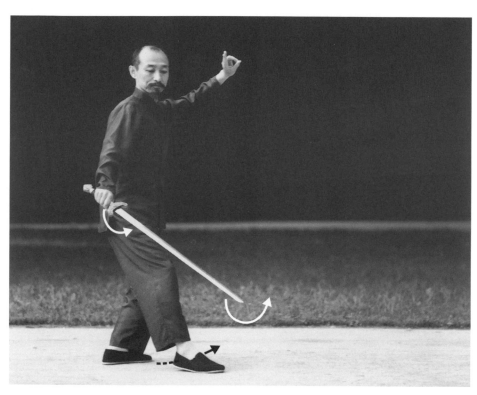

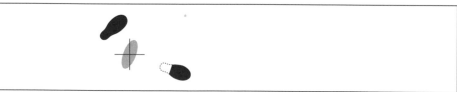

2. Shift your weight further onto your left foot, turn your torso to the right, and place your right leg to the right with the front part of the foot first (toes 30°). As you start turning your torso, turn the sword counterclockwise, and then direct it diagonally downward. Simultaneously, raise the rounded left arm (sword finger).

You are in the position "The Black Dragon Hits with His Tail."

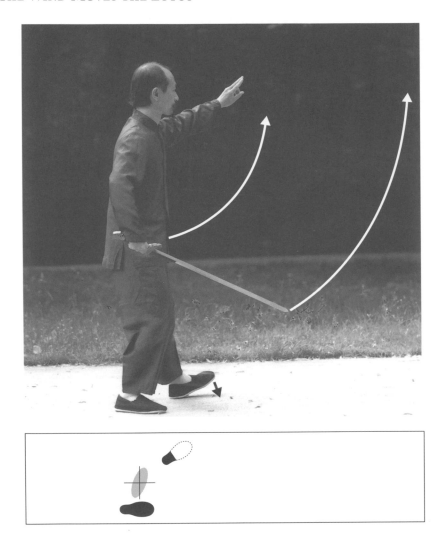

(Not shown): Lift your right leg and place the foot, heel first, about a foot's width SW; the tip of the foot points NW.

1. Shift your weight onto your right foot, turn your torso left, and place your left leg to the SW, heel first (Bow Step). Simultaneously, bend your right arm and turn the sword clockwise until the blade lies flat.

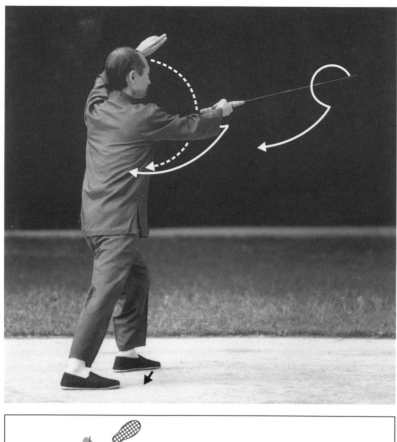

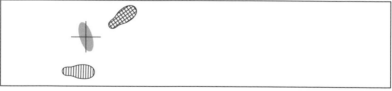

2. Shift your weight onto your left foot and direct the sword diagonally upward. Your left arm remains in a raised position. You are in the position "The Wind Moves the Lotus."

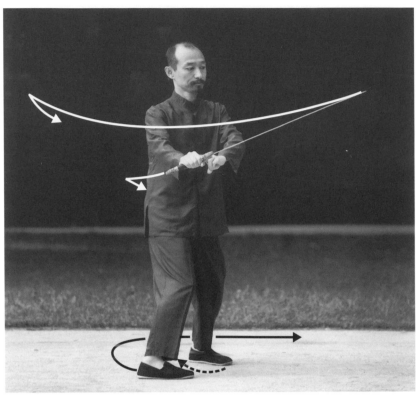

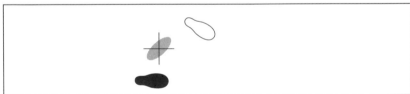

1. Shift your weight onto your right foot, turn your torso right, and turn your left foot on its heel until your toes point NW. Simultaneously, lower your right arm to your body, and turn the sword counterclockwise. At the same time, lower your rounded left arm and point the sword finger at your right wrist.

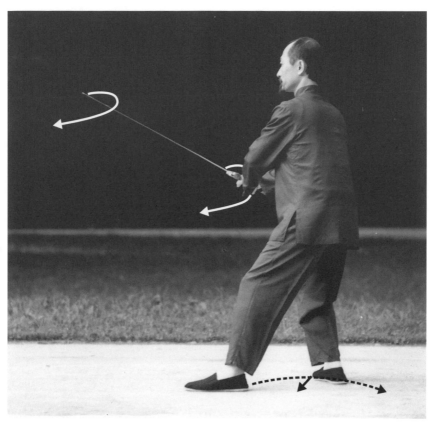

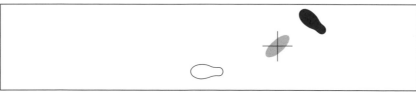

2. Turn your torso further to the right. While doing this, guide your right leg in a large arc over the outside and place it backward, SW, with the front part of the foot first; the toes point SE.

Near the end of shifting your weight onto your right foot, turn your left foot on its heel until your toes point E (Bow Step). Your arms and the sword follow the torso's movement and are directed in front of the right side of your body.

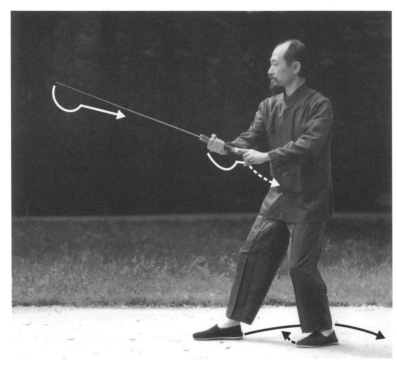

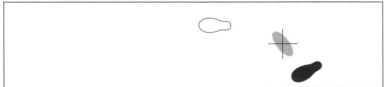

3. (a) Turn your torso left and place your left leg back with the front part of the foot first, the toes pointing NE. While doing this, turn the sword in a small clockwise arc until the back of your hand faces down.

(b) Turn your torso further left and shift your weight onto your left foot. Near the end of the weight shift, turn the heel of your right foot until your toes point E (Bow Step). Direct your arms and the sword, at the same time, in front of the left side of your body. The sword finger remains pointed at your right wrist.

A repetition of "The Lion Shakes His Mane" in the left Bow Step follows (see illustration 2).

A repetition of The Lion Shakes His Mane" in the right Bow Step follows (see illustration 3 (a) and (b)).

You are in the position "The Lion Shakes His Mane."

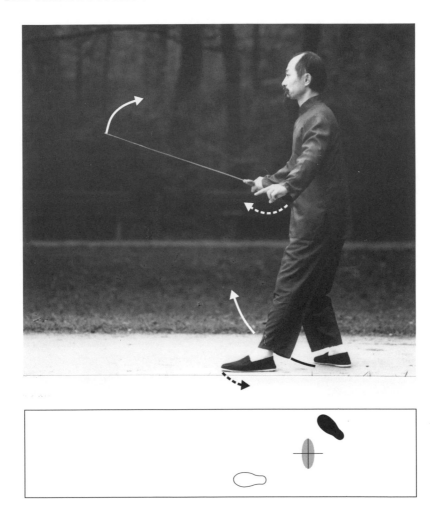

1. (a) Place the right leg backward, with the front part of the foot first. Turn the sword counterclockwise at the same time until the back of your hand faces up.

(b) Shift your weight onto your right foot, turn your torso somewhat to the right and move your arms apart.

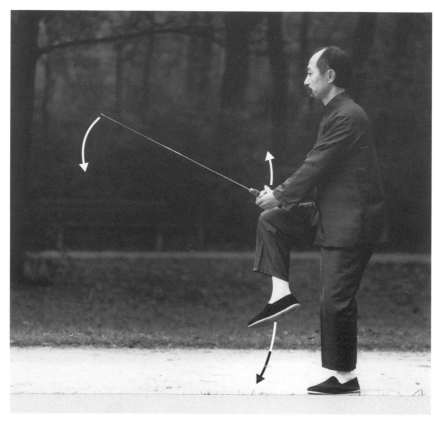

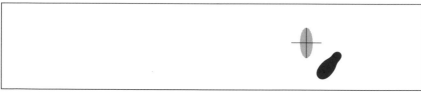

2. (a) Turn the heel of your left foot to the NE.

(b) Shift your weight onto your left foot, lift your right leg, and bring both arms together, making circular arcs from below. While doing this, open the sword finger and place your left hand under your right hand. Simultaneously raise the tip of the sword.

You are in the position "The Tiger Puts His Head Between His Paws."

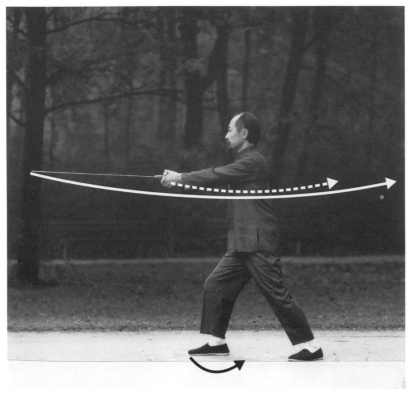

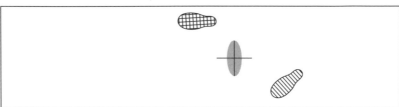

(Not shown): The following movement prepares you for the jump. First lower your right leg and shift your weight onto your right foot. While doing this, lower the tip of the sword, then draw up your left leg (see position 8, "The Clever Cat Catches a Mouse," illustration 2).

(Not shown): Jump from your right leg (foot) onto your left leg. At the same time, lift the blade again (see position 8, "The Clever Cat Catches a Mouse," illustration 3).

1. Slow down the movement and, in the right Bow Step, bring both arms forward.

You are in the position "The Wild Horse Springs over the Mountain Stream."

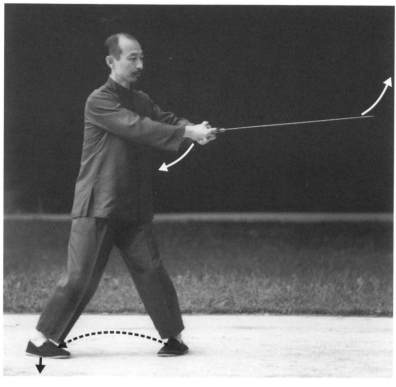

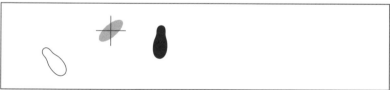

1. Shift your weight onto your left foot. While doing this, turn your torso left and pivot your right foot on its heel until your toes point NW. Your arms and the sword follow the movement of your torso.

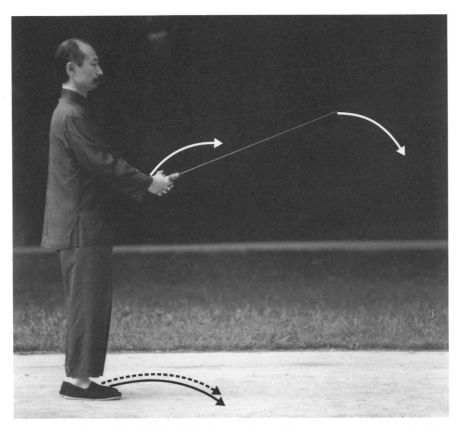

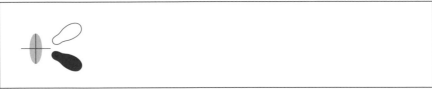

2. (a) Place your right leg a foot's length to the N, with the heel first.

(b) Shift your weight onto your right foot, turn your torso left, and place your left foot next to your right foot. Pull in your arms and the sword slightly to your body (rein in the horse), and raise the tip of the sword a little. You are in the position "Turn Around and Rein In the Horse."

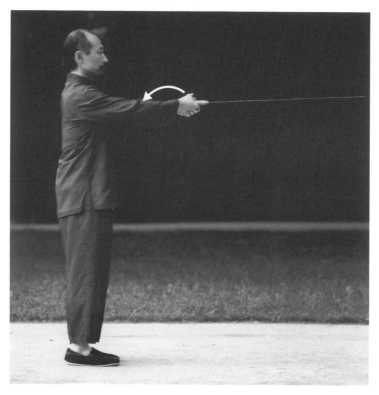

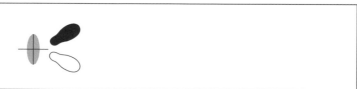

1. Place your left leg forward and then bring your right foot next to your left foot. Direct your arms and the sword upward and forward.

You are in the position "Step Forward—the Compass Needle Points South."

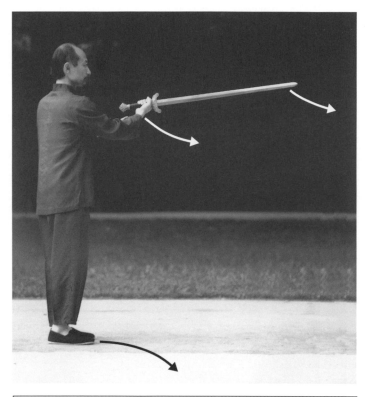

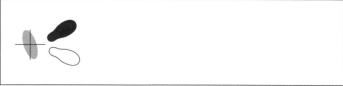

1. Shift your weight completely onto your left foot, bend your left knee somewhat, and turn your torso slightly to the left. While doing this, bring your arms to your body and turn the sword slightly clockwise. Simultaneously, release your left hand from your right hand, turn it a little clockwise, form the sword finger, and direct it at your right wrist.

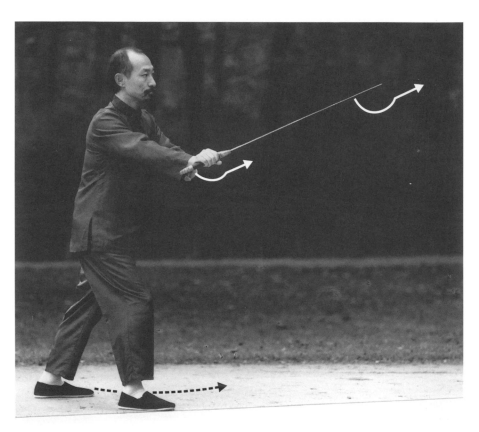

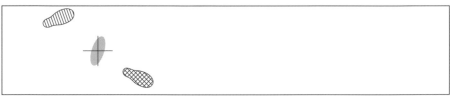

2. Place your right leg forward to the right, heel first (toes 30°). Shift your weight onto your right foot and turn your torso to the right. At the beginning of the movement, direct the sword in a counterclockwise arc until the back of your hand faces up. Along with shifting your weight and turning your torso, guide the sword in front of the right side of your body. The sword finger remains pointed at your right wrist.

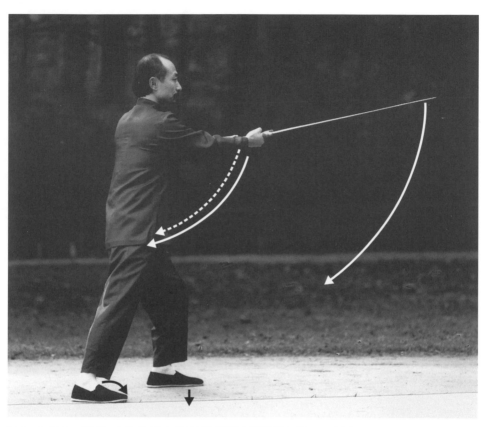

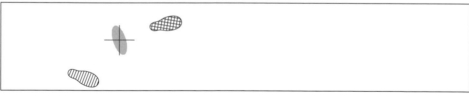

3. (a) Shift your weight completely onto your right foot (release in the groin fold) and turn your torso somewhat to the right. Turn the sword at the same time in a clockwise arc until the back of your hand faces down.

(b) Place your left leg forward to the left, heel first (toes 30°). Shift your weight onto your left foot; turn your torso to the left at the same time. Along with this, guide the sword in front of the left side of your body. The sword finger remains pointed at your right wrist. You are in the position "Shake Off the Dust in the Wind."

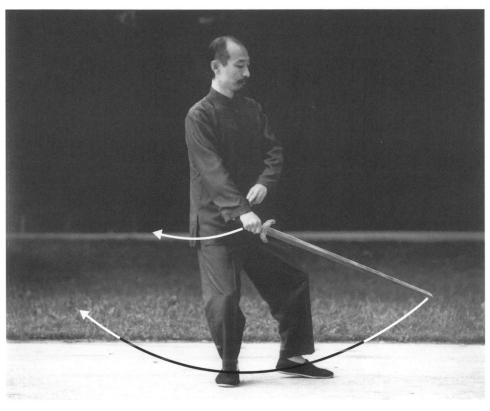

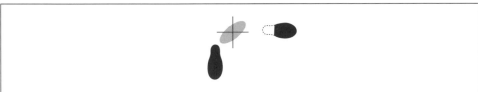

1. (a) Shift your weight completely onto the left foot. Lift the right leg and place it to the N, heel first.

(b) Shift your weight onto your right foot; while doing this, turn your torso right, and place your left leg with the front part of the foot N. Lower your arms and the sword. Bring the blade of the sword into a standing position through a small counterclockwise turn.

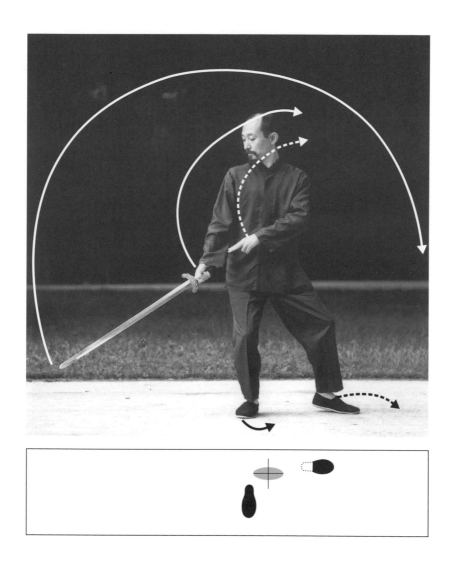

2. Turn your torso further to the right. At the same time, turn the sword clockwise until the blade is standing again and the tip of the sword points E.

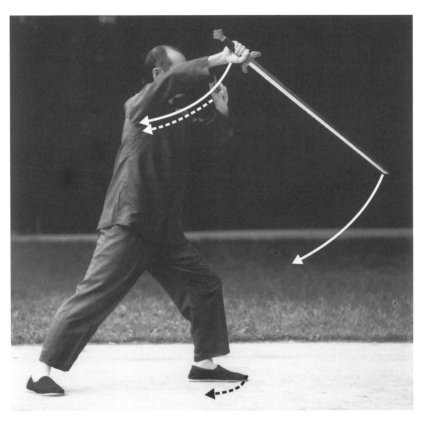

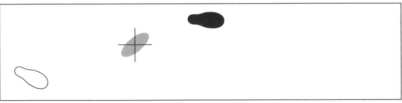

3. (a) Slightly stretch your right leg, turn your torso somewhat to the left, and lift your left leg. Simultaneously, begin lifting the sword in an outward arc.

(b) Turn your torso further to the left and place your left leg forward to the W, heel first, toes pointing W (Bow Step). Lift the sword further; the sword finger remains pointed at your right wrist.

(c) Shift your weight onto your left foot; at the same time, direct the sword forward, further along the arc—with the same motion as in pushing something along (send the boat downstream). Near the end of the movement, direct the tip of the sword somewhat downward. The sword finger remains pointed at your right wrist.

Note: Don't take the sword over your head! Reduce the size of the arc by bending your right arm.

You are in the position "Send the Boat Downstream."

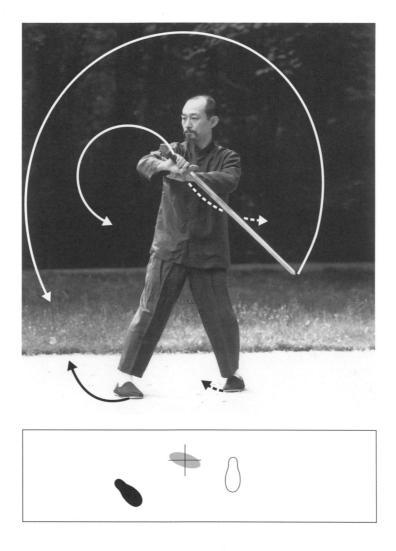

1. Shift your weight onto your right foot, turn your torso right, and turn your left foot on its heel until your toes point N. Your arms and the sword lower somewhat while accompanying the turning of your torso and the shifting of your weight.

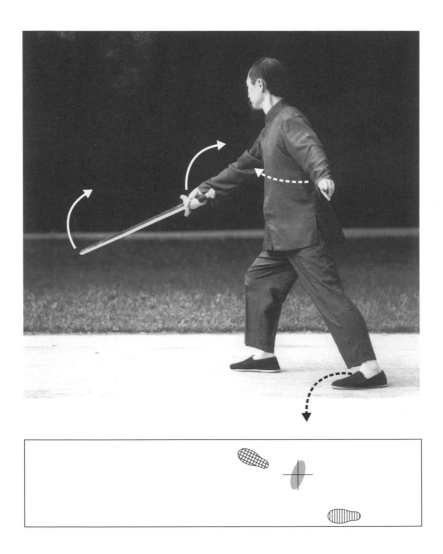

2. (a) Shift your weight onto your left foot. Turn your torso right and place your right foot to the NE, heel first (toes pointing NE).

(b) Shift your weight onto your right foot; at the same time, turn your torso further right and pivot your left foot on its heel until your toes point E (Bow Step). Simultaneously, guide the sword in an arc forward from above, moving SE; the blade of the sword stands. Your left arm (sword finger) extends to the N.

Note: Extend your right arm only near the end of the movement so that the arc won't be too large. Don't move the sword over your head.

You are in the position "The Shooting Star Follows the Moon."

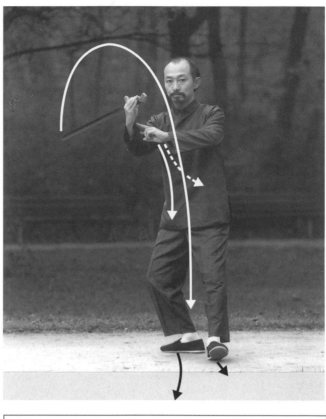

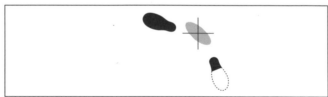

1. (a) Shift your weight completely onto your right foot.

(b) Turn your torso left and lift your left leg. At the same time, turn the sword clockwise.

(c) Place your left leg forward, heel first, toes pointing NW. While doing this, lift the sword by bending your right arm and pull it to the side of your body. Bend your left arm so that the sword finger again points at your right wrist.

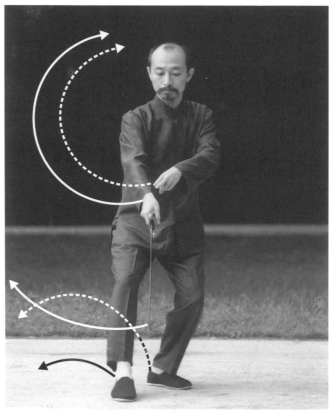

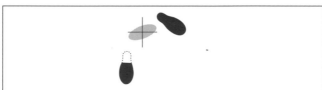

2. Shift your weight onto your left leg, turn your torso further to the left, and place your right leg forward with the front part of the foot pointing N (Step of the Fishing Horse). Simultaneously, guide the sword in a forward arc in front of your body; the blade of the sword stands. The sword finger is pointed at your right wrist.

You are in the position "The Heavenly Horse Flies Through the Air."

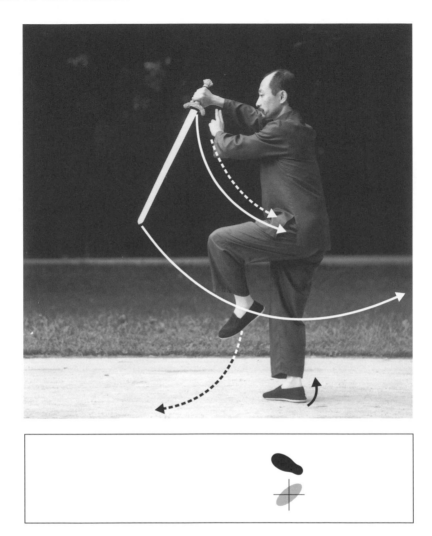

1. (a) Turn your torso right, and place your right leg to the E, heel first, toes pointing SE. At the same time, turn your arms and the sword somewhat counterclockwise.

(b) Shift your weight onto your right foot. Lift your left leg by slightly stretching your right leg. Simultaneously, guide your arms and the sword upward in front of your body. The sword finger remains pointed at your right wrist. You are in the position "Move the Curtain."

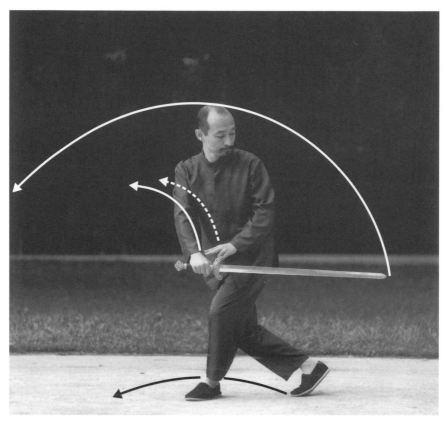

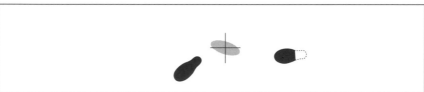

1. Place your left leg forward to the E, heel first, toes pointing NE. Shift your weight onto your left foot and bend your knee. Simultaneously, turn your torso to the left and pick up the heel of your right foot and point it W. This is accompanied by lowering the sword with a standing blade and moving it backward to the W, passing it by your left side. The sword finger remains pointed at your right wrist.

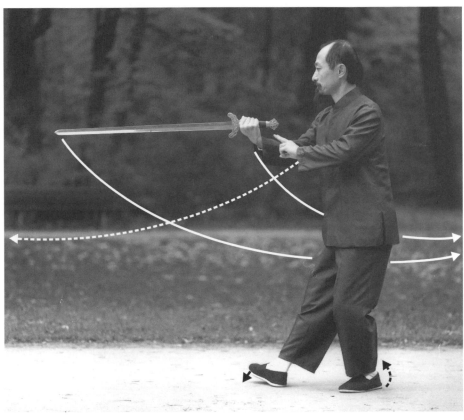

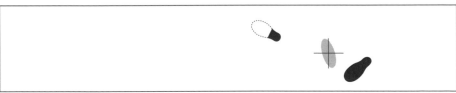

2. Turn your torso right, slightly stretching your left leg, and place your right leg forward E, on the heel, the toes pointing SSE. Along with this, lift the sword with a standing blade past your left side (cartwheel), and bring it horizontally in front of your body. The sword finger remains pointed at your right wrist.

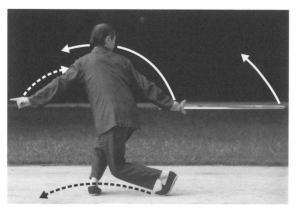

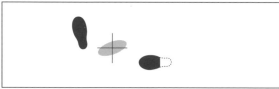

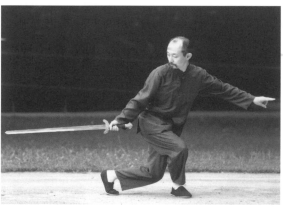

Front View

3. Shift your weight onto your right foot. At the same time, bend your right knee and turn the torso W. While doing this, lower the sword past your right side and direct it backward; at the end of the movement, put the blade in a standing position after a small turn counterclockwise. Your left arm (sword finger) points forward.

Note: The sequence of movements described here in illustrations 2 and 3 are performed continuously without pause.

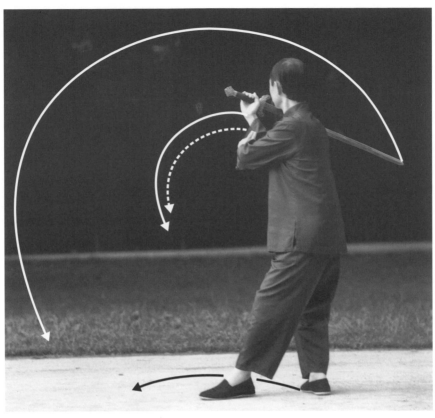

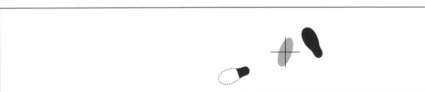

4. Shift your weight completely onto your right foot and stretch your right leg. Turn your torso left, and place your left leg forward, heel first, toes pointing NE. At the same time, turn the sword slightly clockwise (the tip of the sword remains pointed to the W), then lift it with a standing blade on the right side of your body. Simultaneously, bend your left arm and point the sword finger at your right wrist again.

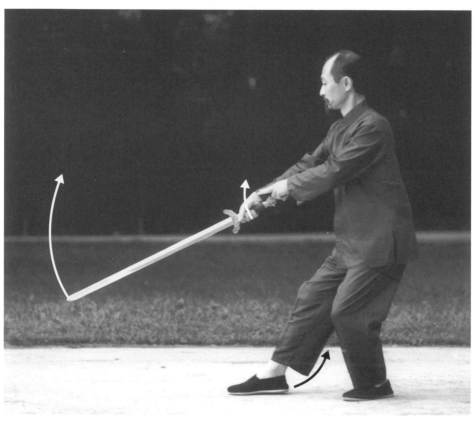

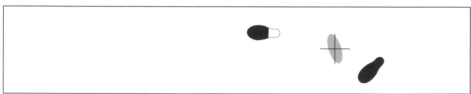

5. Shift your weight onto your left foot, turn your torso left, and place your right leg forward E with the front part of the foot, your toes pointing E (Step of the Fishing Horse). Simultaneously, lower the sword with a standing blade from above in front of your body. The sword finger remains pointed at your right wrist.

You are in the position "The Sword Circles Like a Cartwheel—Left and Right."

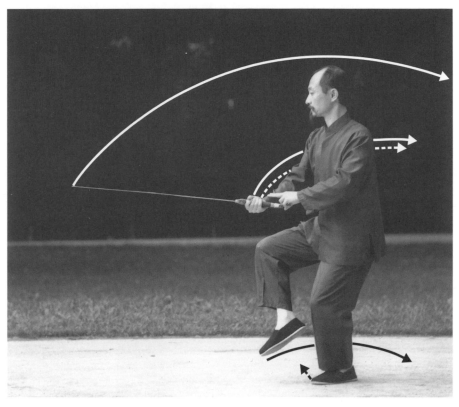

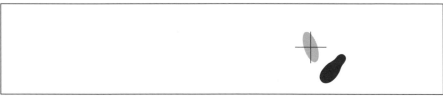

1. Stretch your left leg somewhat; at the same time, lift your right leg and turn your torso a little to the left. Simultaneously, bend your right arm and turn the sword in a small clockwise arc until the blade lies flat; raise the tip of the sword while doing so (the tip of the sword remains pointed to the E). The sword finger points at your right wrist.

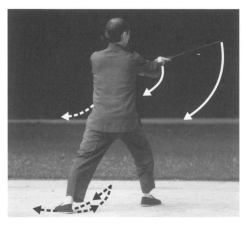

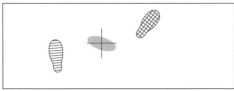

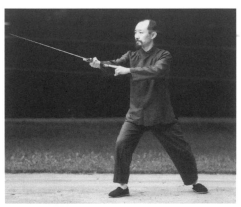

Front View

2. (a) Turn your torso right and place your right leg to the SW, heel first, the toes pointing SW.

(b) Shift your weight onto your right foot, turn your torso right at the same time, and pivot your left foot on its heel until your toes point S (Bow Step). Your arms and the sword follow the movement of your torso and are directed diagonally up to the SW.

You are in the position "The Mythical Bird Spreads One Wing."

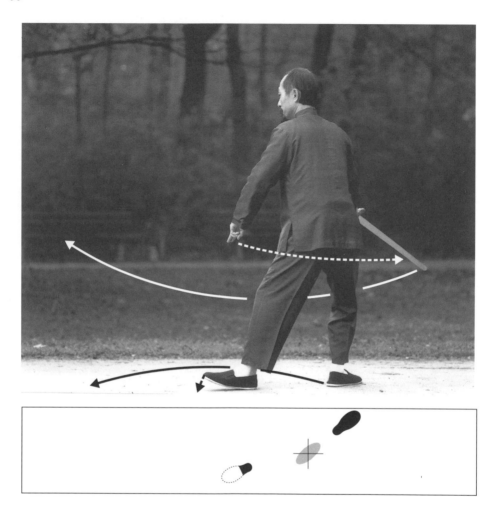

(Not shown): Shift your weight completely onto your right foot and lift your left leg.

1. Turn your torso to the left and place your left leg to the NE, heel first, toes pointing NE. At the same time, turn the sword counterclockwise until the blade stands; lower both arms (the tip of the sword remains pointing to the SW).

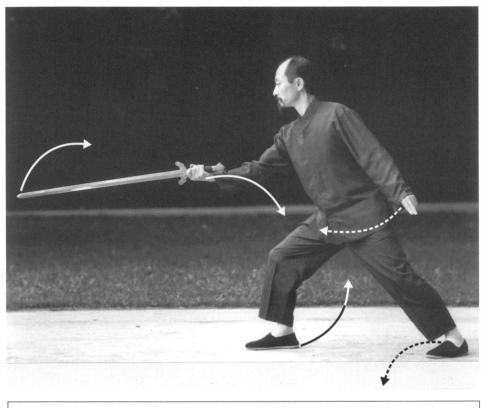

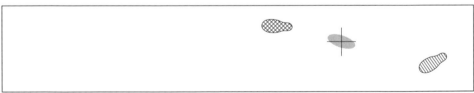

2. (a) Shift your weight onto your left foot, turn your torso left, and place your right leg forward to the E, heel first (Bow Step). While doing this, lower the sword further and turn it slightly clockwise, directing it forward from below.

(b) Without pausing, shift your weight onto your right foot and turn your torso further to the left. At the same time, guide the sword in front of your body, continuing the arc. While doing so, bring the blade into a standing position and point the tip of the sword to the E. Guide your left arm (sword finger) backward while turning your torso during Steps 1 and 2.

You are in the position "Lift the Moon from the Bottom of the Sea."

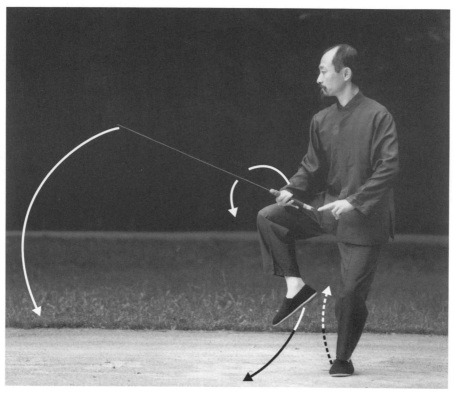

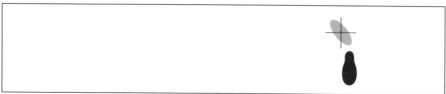

(Not shown): Shift your weight completely onto your right foot. Lift your left leg and place it about a foot's width forward with the front part of the foot first, toes pointing N.

1. Shift the weight onto the left foot. Turn your torso somewhat to the left, and pull in your right leg. Simultaneously, direct the sword in front of

the left side of your body and, while doing so, turn it slightly counterclockwise until the blade lies flat; raise the tip of the sword. At the same time, direct your left arm (sword finger) forward, and point the sword finger at the sword's knob.

You are in the position "Embrace the Moon."

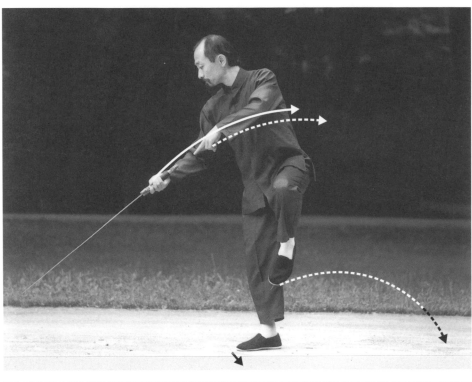

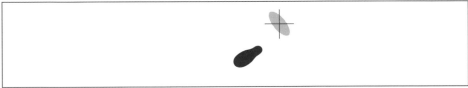

1. (a) Place your right leg forward, heel first (toes 30°).

(b) Shift your weight onto your right foot. At the same time, slightly stretch your right leg and bend your torso a little forward; direct the sword downward by stretching your arm. Simultaneously, lift your left leg. The sword finger is pointed at your right wrist.

You are in the position "The Demon Looks into the Water."

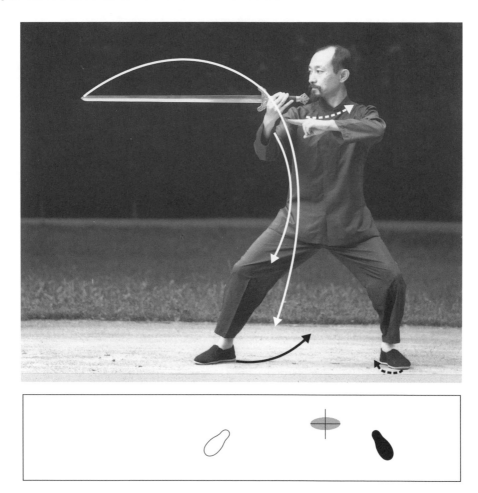

1. (a) Place your left leg backward to the W, heel first (toes 30°).

(b) Shift your weight onto your left foot and bend your knee. At the same time, turn your torso somewhat to the left and pivot your right foot on its heel until your toes point to the NE. Simultaneously, bend your right elbow, which pulls the sword to your body and raises the blade into a standing position. The sword finger remains pointed at your right wrist.

You are in the position "The Rhinoceros Looks at the Moon."

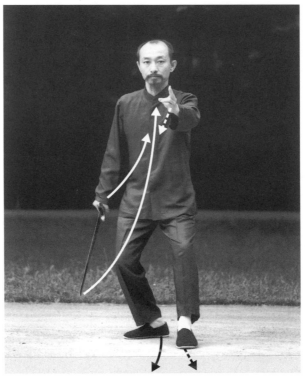

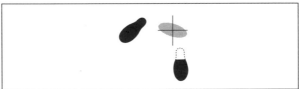

(Not shown): Shift your weight completely onto your left foot, and place your right leg backward with the front part of the foot first, toes pointing NE.

1. Shift the weight onto the right foot, turn the torso right, and place the left leg about a foot's width right with the front part of the foot (Step of the Fishing Horse). Simultaneously lower the sword to your right side with a counterclockwise arc until the blade stands. At the same time, stretch your left arm out forward; the sword finger points forward and up.

You are in the position "Shoot the Swallow."

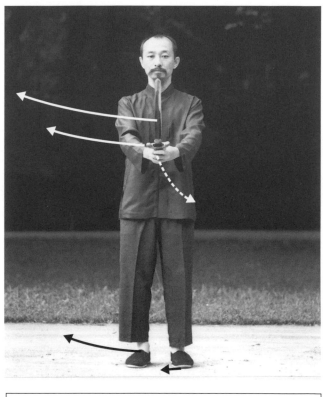

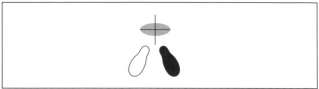

1. (a) Place your left leg forward, heel first (toes 30°).

(b) Shift your weight onto your left foot and place your right foot next to your left foot (toes 30°). Simultaneously turn the sword clockwise and direct it forward and up in front of the body (the tip of the sword points up). At the same time, lower your left arm, open the sword finger, and place your left hand under your right hand.

(For side view, see illustration 42, "The White Monkey Offers Fruit," Step 1 a and b.)

You are in the position "The White Monkey Offers Fruit."

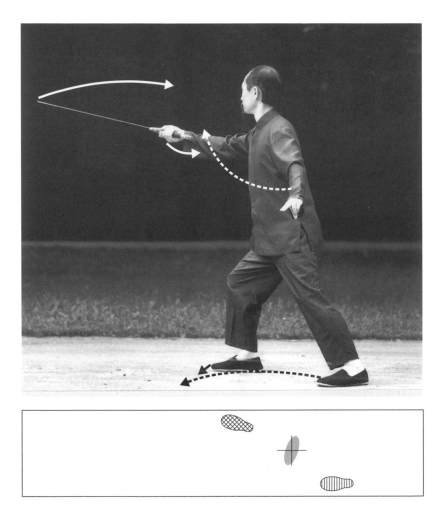

(Not shown): Shift your weight completely onto your left foot and turn your torso a little to the left. While doing so, direct the sword somewhat left; simultaneously, release your left hand from your right and, turning it clockwise, form the sword finger. Your right arm moves under your left.

1. Place your right leg in an outward arc, heel first to the SE, toes pointing SE. Shift your weight onto your right foot, turn your torso right, and pivot your left foot on its heel until your toes point E (Bow Step). Along with this, direct the sword diagonally upward to the right; your left hand forms the sword finger and points N.

You are in the position "The Phoenix Spreads Its Wings."

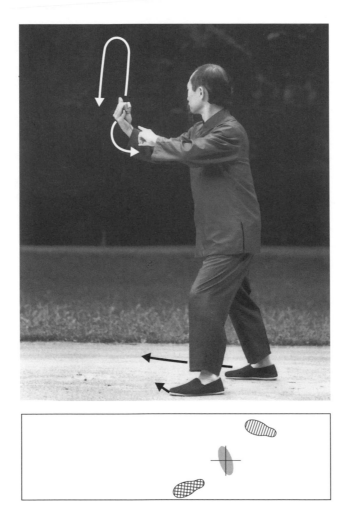

1. (a) Shift your weight completely onto your right foot, and place your left leg forward left, heel first (toes 30°).

(b) Without a pause, shift your weight onto your left foot, turn your torso slightly to the left, and pivot your right foot on its heel (toes 30°). While doing so, first turn the sword slightly clockwise and then pull it to the left in front of your body (the standing blade is held horizontally; the tip of the sword points S. Along with shifting your weight and turning your torso, bend your left arm and point the sword finger at your right wrist.

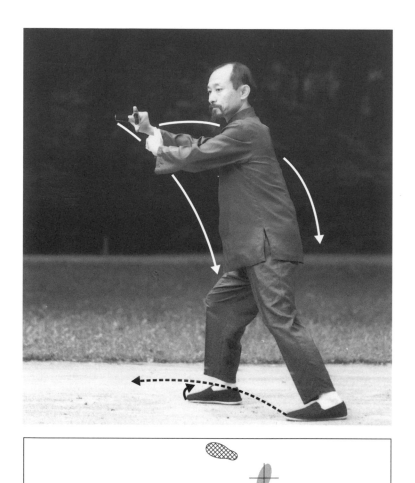

2. (a) Shift your weight completely onto your right foot (release in the groin fold). Simultaneously, lower both arms somewhat.

(b) Place your right leg forward to the right, heel first (toes 30°); turn your torso slightly right; and by bending your elbow, draw a circular arc downward to the left with the sword.

(c) Shift your weight onto your right foot. Turn your torso further to the right and, while doing so, pull the sword to the right in front of your body; the standing blade is held horizontally. (the tip of the sword remains pointed to the N).

You are in the position "Halt—Left and Right—with Step."

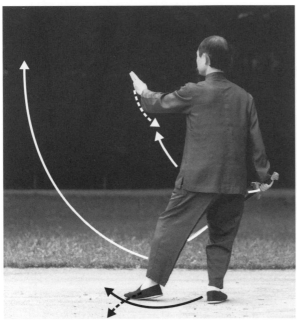

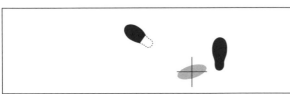

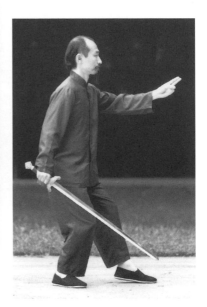

Side View

1. (a) Turn your torso slightly to the right; at the same time, direct the front part of your right foot to the right until your toes point S.

(b) Shift your weight completely onto your right foot; while doing so, place your left leg forward to the SE, with the front part of the foot first. Lower the sword, following an arc, to your right side until the blade stands. Direct your left arm (sword finger) forward and upward to the SE.

You are in the position "Shoot the Wild Goose."

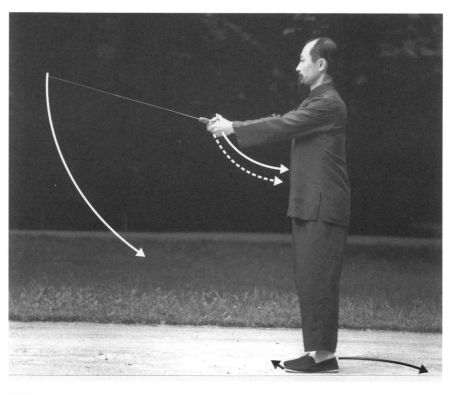

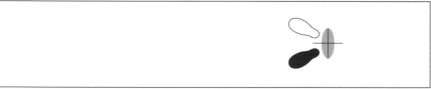

1. (a) Shift your weight completely onto your right foot, turn your torso to the left, and place your left leg forward to the left, heel first (toes 30°).

(b) Shift your weight onto your left foot and place your right foot next to the left foot (toes 30°). Simultaneously, turn the sword clockwise and, while bending your right elbow, direct it in front of your body forward and upward until the blade lies flat. At the same time, direct the tip of the sword upward, shift your weight onto your left foot, lower your left arm, open the sword finger, and place your left hand under your right hand.

You are in the position "The White Monkey Offers Fruit."

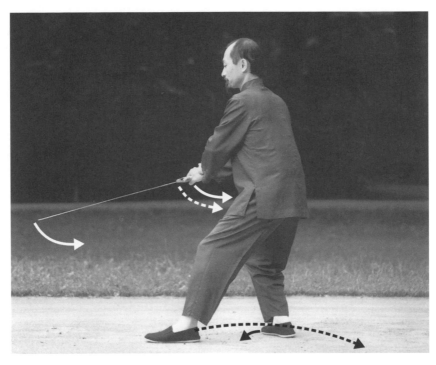

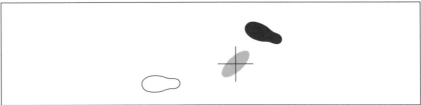

1. (a) Shift your weight completely onto your left foot and turn your torso a little left. Simultaneously, lower your arms somewhat and pull them to your body. While doing so, turn the sword a little clockwise; release your left hand from your right hand, turning it clockwise to form the sword finger; and point it at your right wrist.

(b) Turn your torso right and place your right leg backward to the right. Turn the sword at the same time in a counterclockwise arc until the back of your hand faces up.

(c) Without pausing, shift your weight onto your right foot, turn your torso further to the right, and, finally, turn the front part of your left foot until the toes point E (Bow Step). At the same time, while turning your torso and shifting your weight, direct the sword downward in front of the right side of your body. The sword finger remains pointed at your right wrist.

Note: "Scatter Flowers—Left and Right" is similar to "The Lion Shakes His Mane." In the performance of the former, the sword stays on the same level, and the tip of the sword points a little upward. In "Scatter Flowers—Left and Right," the tip of the sword is down and the sword sinks progressively downward during the sequence of the movement.

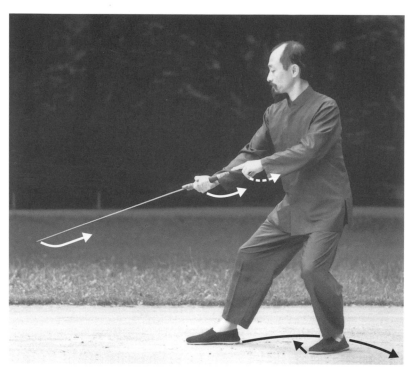

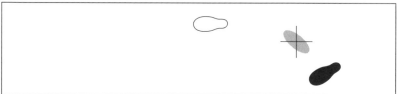

2. (a) Shift your weight completely onto your right foot and turn the sword in a clockwise arc until the back of your hand faces down.

(b) Turn your torso left and place your left leg backward with the front part of the foot first (toes pointing NE).

(c) Shift your weight onto your left foot; while doing so, turn your torso further to the left and finally turn the front part of your right foot inward until the toes point E (Bow Step). Along with shifting your weight and turning your torso, direct the sword in front of the left side of

your body. The sword finger remains pointed at your right wrist.

Followed by the repetition of:
"Scatter Flowers—Left and Right" in a left Bow Step (see illustration 1 a–c).
"Scatter Flowers—Left and Right" in a right Bow Step (see illustration 2 a–c).
"Scatter Flowers—Left and Right" in a left Bow Step (see illustration 1 a–c).

With the last repetition, you are in the position "Scatter Flowers—Left and Right."

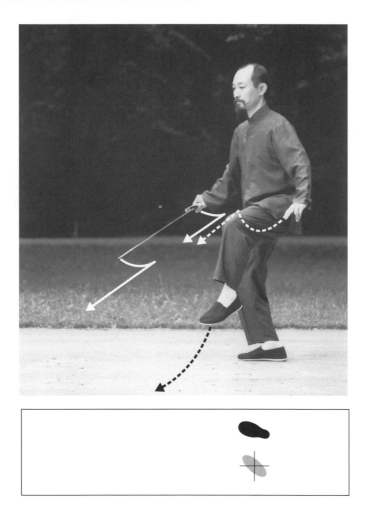

1. Turn your torso left, lift your left leg, and direct your left arm (sword finger) to the left side of your body.

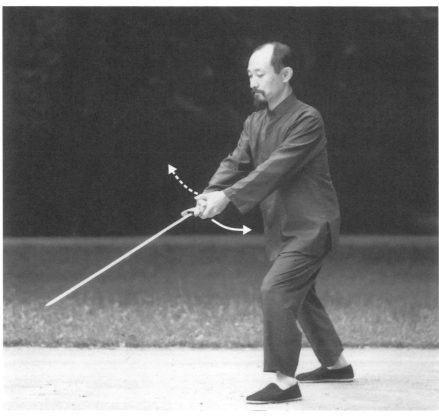

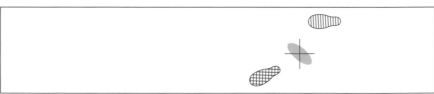

2. (a) Place your left leg forward to the NE, heel first, toes pointing NE.

(b) Shift your weight onto your left foot and then pivot your right foot inward until your toes point E (Bow Step). Along with the weight shift, bring your arms together; while doing so, turn the sword clockwise until the blade lies flat.

Open your left hand, turn it counterclockwise, and place it under your right hand. Toward the end of the movement, direct the sword downward and forward.

You are in the position "Fair Lady Threads the Shuttle."

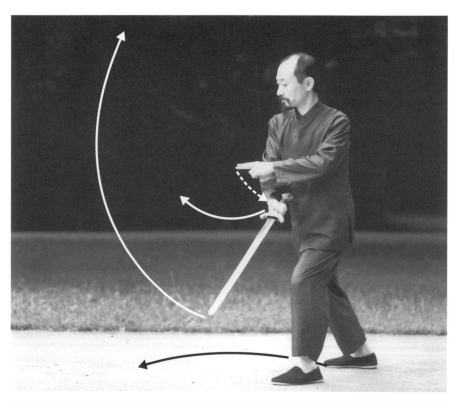

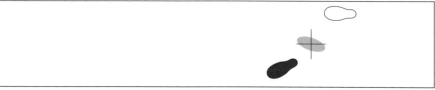

1. Shift your weight completely onto your left foot; turn your torso slightly to the left. Along with this, direct the sword to the left, release your left hand from your right hand, turn it clockwise, and form the sword finger. Your right arm moves under your left arm.

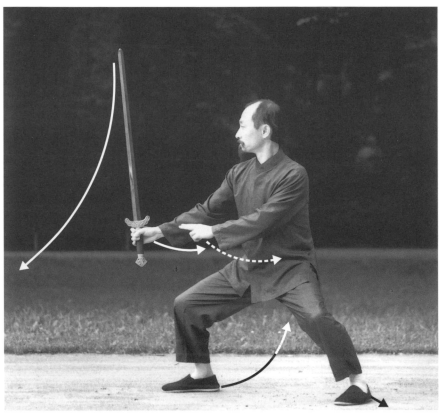

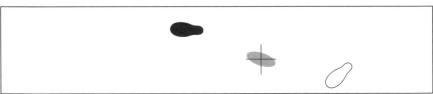

2. (a) Place your right leg forward to the E, heel first, toes pointing E (Bow Step).

(b) Shift your weight onto your right foot, crouch down, and direct the sword with a standing blade from below, forward and up. The sword finger points at your right wrist.

You are in the position "The White Tiger Hits with His Tail."

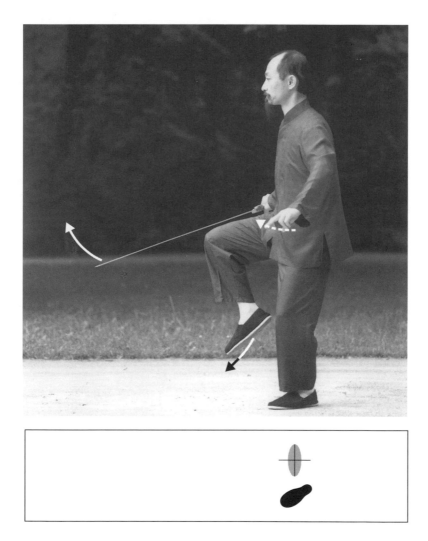

1. (a) Turn the heel of your left foot somewhat backward to the W.

(b) Shift your weight onto your left foot; stretch your left leg at the same time and pull up your right leg. Simultaneously, turn your torso somewhat to the right and move your arms apart. At the same time, turn the sword counterclockwise and, with the blade in a lying position, direct it to your right side.

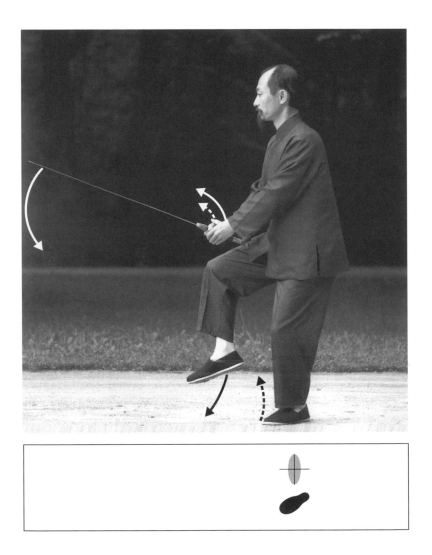

2. Stretch your left leg a little. Bring both arms together in circular arcs from below. At the same time, turn the sword clockwise and raise the tip. Open your left hand (sword finger) and place it under your right hand.

You are in the position "The Tiger Puts His Head Between His Paws."

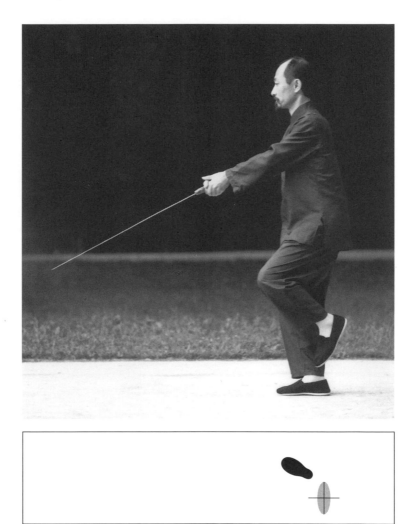

1. Prepare to make a jump: first lower your right leg, shift your weight onto your right foot, then pull up your left leg and, while doing so, lower the blade.

(Not shown): The jump occurs from the right leg (foot) onto the left leg; at the same time, the blade is lifted again (see position 8, "The Clever Cat Catches a Mouse," illustration 3).

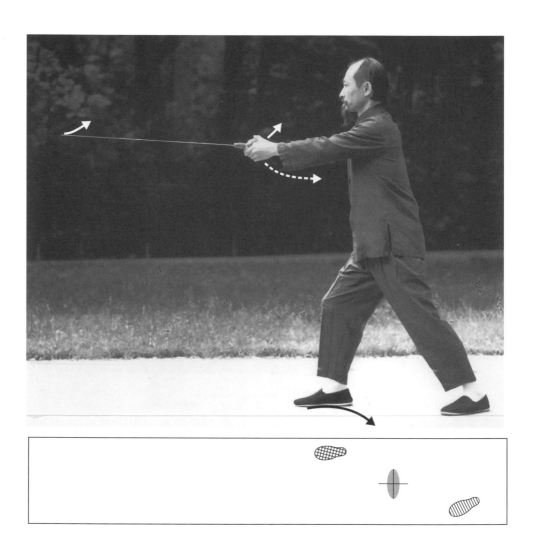

2. Slow down the movement in a right Bow Step and guide both arms forward.

You are in the position "The Carp Jumps Through the Dragon Gate."

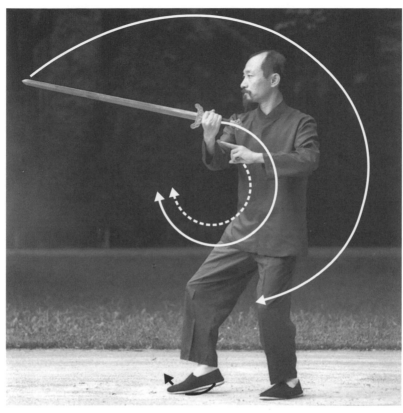

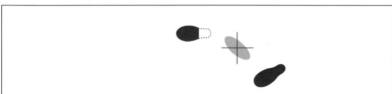

1. Shift your weight completely onto your left foot. Turn your torso to the left, lift your right leg slightly, and place it with the front part of the foot backward; your toes remain pointed to the E (Step of the Fishing Horse). Simultaneously, turn the sword slightly clockwise until the blade stands. At the same time, release your left hand from your right hand, turn the back of the hand upward, form the sword finger, and point at your right wrist.

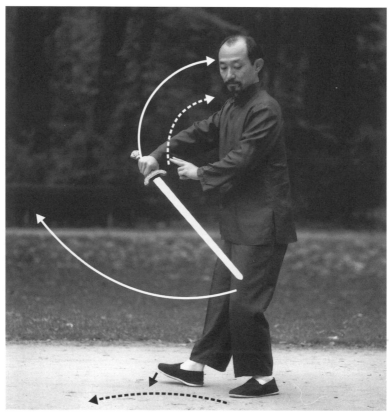

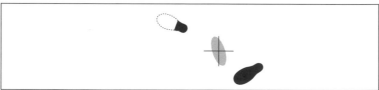

(Not shown): Turn your torso further to the left, and guide the sword, with a standing blade, backward in a large arc. At the same time, lift your right leg.

2. Turn your torso slightly right and place your right foot forward with the heel first and the toes pointing SE. While doing this, direct the sword forward, continuing the arc past the left side of your body. The sword finger remains pointed at your right wrist.

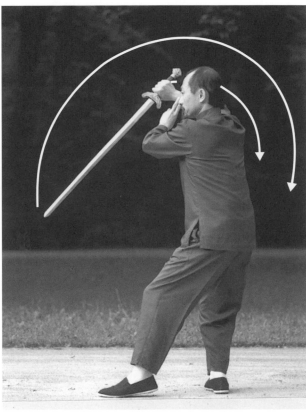

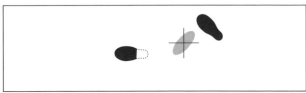

3. Shift your weight onto your right foot, turn your torso right, and place your left leg forward to the E on the front part of the foot, toes pointing E (Step of the Fishing Horse). Along with this, raise the sword in front of your body from below. The sword finger remains pointed at your right wrist.

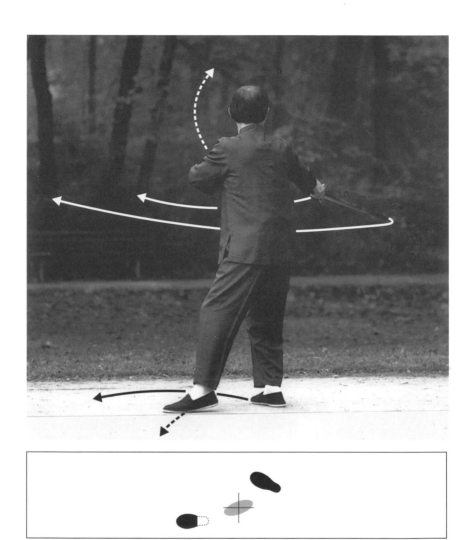

4. Turn your torso to the right and lower the sword SW with a standing blade. The sword finger remains pointed at your right wrist.

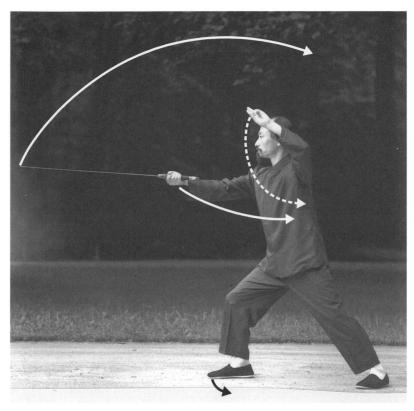

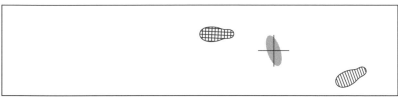

5. (a) Shift your weight completely onto your right foot, turn your torso to the left, and place your left leg forward left, heel first, toes pointing NE. At the same time, lower the sword somewhat and turn it clockwise.

(b) Shift your weight onto your left foot, turn your torso further to the left, and place your right leg forward to the E, heel first, toes pointing E (Bow Step). The sword follows the movement of your torso and, by bending your right elbow, comes forward to the E.

(c) Shift your weight onto your right foot and turn your torso further to the left. While doing this, guide the sword forward with a lying blade to the E. Lift your rounded left arm (sword finger).

You are in the position "The Black Dragon Twines Around a Column."

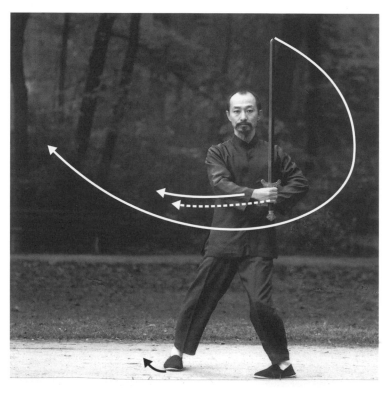

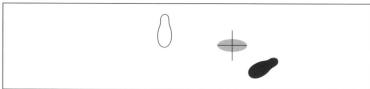

1. Shift your weight onto your left foot; at the same time, turn your torso left, and pivot your right foot on its heel until your toes point N. Simultaneously, direct the sword, by bending your right arm, in front of the left side of your body, bringing it into a perpendicular position. Lower your left arm and point the sword finger at your right wrist.

You are in the position "The Holy Man Points Out the Way."

Note: In a well-known version of this position, the left hand is open and in front of the right hand.

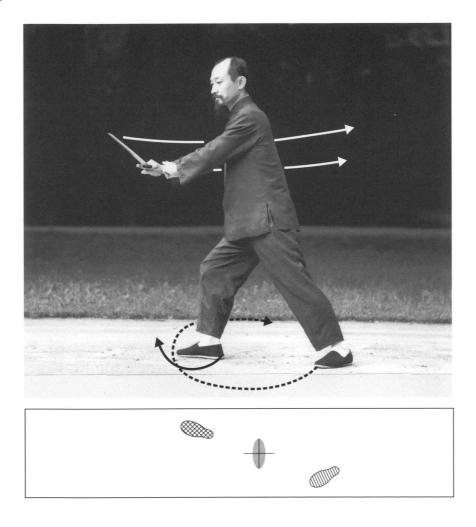

1. Shift your weight onto your right foot, turn your torso to the right, and pivot your right foot on its heel until your toes point SE. Simultaneously, move the sword counterclockwise and bring the blade into a lying position. The sword finger remains pointed at your right wrist.

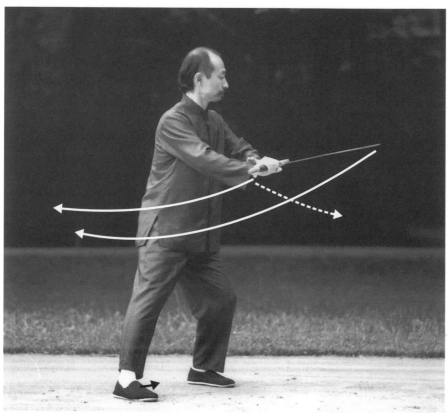

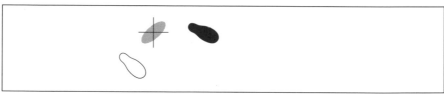

2. (a) Shift your weight completely onto your right foot. At the same time, turn your torso further to the right; lift your left leg; and, moving in a large outward arc to the SW, set it down, heel first. Your arms and the sword follow the movement without changing their position.

(b) Shift your weight onto your left foot, turn your torso further right, and pivot on the front part of your right foot. Your arms and the sword follow the movement of your torso.

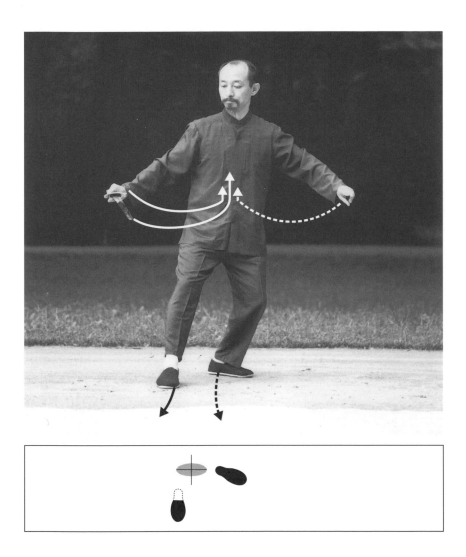

3. Turn the heel of your right foot further left until your toes point forward N (Step of the Fishing Horse). While doing so, turn your torso further to the right and move your arms apart.

You are in the position "The Wind Sweeps Away the Plum Blossoms."

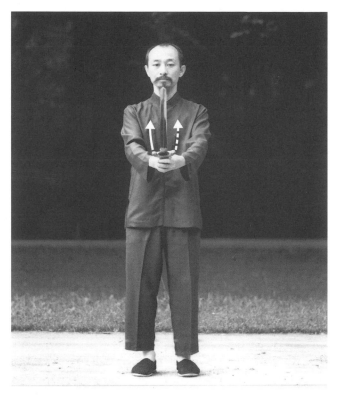

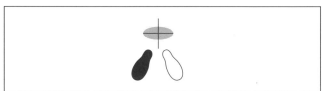

(Not shown): Lift your right leg and place it forward, heel first, toes pointed somewhat outward.

1. Shift your weight onto your right foot and place your left foot forward, toes pointed somewhat outward. Bring your arms together, forming arcs from below. At the same time, turn the sword clockwise and place your left hand (open the sword finger) under your right hand.

You are in the position "The Tiger Puts His Head Between His Paws."

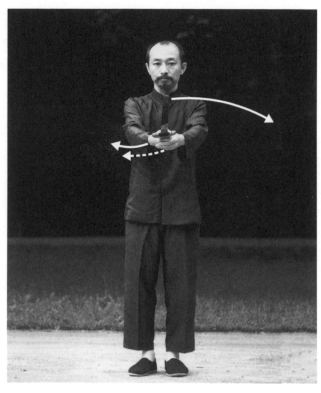

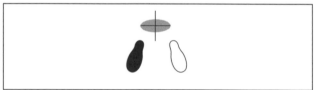

1. Bring your arms and the sword forward. (For side view, see position 25 "Step Forward—the Compass Needle Points South.")

You are in the position, "Step Forward—the Compass Needle Points South."

Note: The position "The Tiger Puts His Head Between His Paws" moves directly into the position "Step Forward—the Compass Needle Points South."

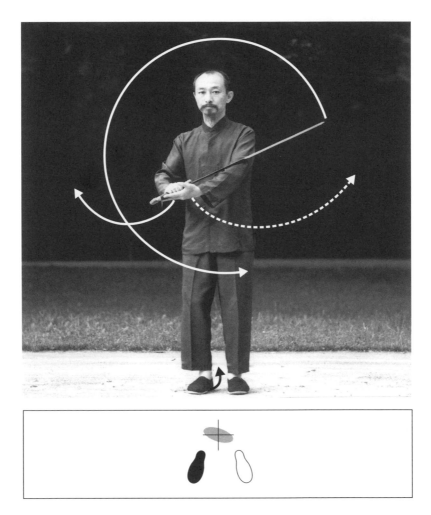

1. Turn your torso slightly to the right and bring your arms somewhat closer to your body. While doing so, turn the sword counterclockwise and guide it to your left arm. The right hand places the sword into the left hand.

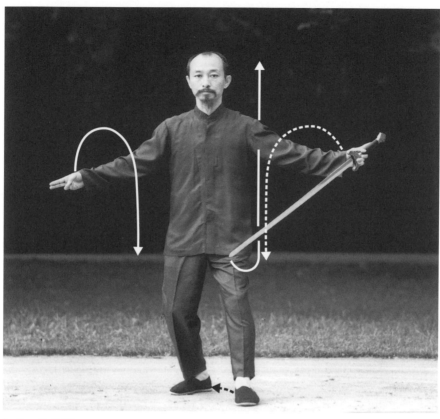

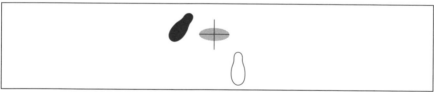

2. (a) Shift your weight onto your left foot and place your right leg back, with the front part of the foot first (toes 30°). Simultaneously, lower your arms and move them apart, raise the tip of the sword, and form the sword finger with your right hand.

(b) Shift your weight onto your right foot. Move your arms outward and lift them up. At the same time, lower the sword in front of your body.

Note: This movement progresses in reverse of position 1 "Awaken the Ch'i at the Beginning"; see illustration 2.

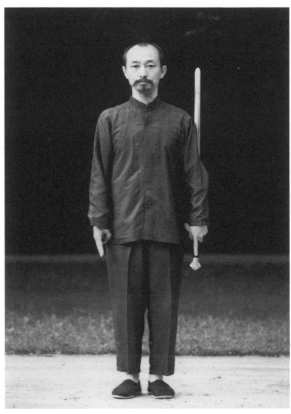

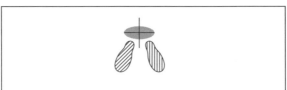

3. Shift your weight completely onto your right foot and place your left foot next to the right foot. Simultaneously, lower your arms from above in arcs to the sides of your body. At the same time, guide the sword behind your lowered left arm.

You are in the position "Turn the Sword over and Return to the Beginning Position."

The performance of the sword form takes about three to five minutes.

A Preface from Chen Wei-Ming's book
The T'ai Chi Sword Fight*

The I Ging says that Taoist knowledge can only be passed on to certain people. That explains the difficulties in conveying Tao at all. With the internal martial arts, there is a similar situation.

In the capital city of Peking, I heard about master Yang Cheng-Fu from Guang Ping. I felt a great admiration for him due to his extraordinary ability in the martial arts. When I asked people who knew him, they all told me, without exception, that I had absolutely no chance to be taught by him. Even his students told me this. When I met master Yang personally, I discovered that he was very accessible and open, that what was said about him was not true. In many publications, similar things were written about master Yang, which is very regrettable since it just isn't the truth.

Before this book, *The T'ai Chi Sword Fight*, I published the book, *T'ai Chi Boxing*; both refer to the teachings of master Yang, and their publication fulfills the wish of master Yang.

The T'ai Chi sword form follows the same principles as the other forms of T'ai Chi Ch'uan and, oriented on these principles, has its own method of application.

In addition to master Yang, I learned T'ai Chi sword from General Li Chin-Lin. I had heard that he was an exceptional sword fighter. Rumors said that he studied with a highly talented teacher. Sun Lu-Tang made a similar remark.

When General Li was staying in Shanghai, I went to meet him. He was very friendly and generously introduced me to the art of the fighting application of the T'ai Chi sword. Moreover, I had the impression that his hip and leg work were very similar to the Push Hands of T'ai Chi Ch'uan and that he practiced the "listening energy," as in T'ai Chi Ch'uan. I hadn't learned any such application of sword fighting from master Yang. General Li's sword isn't constantly in contact with that of his partner, he removes his from the other one. That was really Wu Tan-T'ai Chi sword. With what I learned from master Yang and, in addition, from General Li, I completed my knowledge of the essence and the use of T'ai Chi sword. I would like to publish something about the application of the sword techniques when I have acquired more experience.

* Translation of the original Chinese title of Chen Wei-Ming's book; the preface is shortened, it has been translated into German in 1994 for the German edition. Chen Wei-Ming's book is now available under the title *Taiji Sword and Other Writings*, translated by Barbara Davis, North Atlantic Books.

An Interview*

QUESTION: The T'ai Chi sword form is practiced with a weapon. For me, this brings up the question, "Isn't it contrary to the spiritual claims of T'ai Chi Ch'uan, its meditative practice, releasing, and so on?"

ANSWER: I also used to think in a similar way. However, with increased practicing, this has changed. To begin with, there is not such a great difference between the sword form, the short form, and the long form as one would think. The sword form follows the same principles as the others; it contains the same steps (Bow Step, Step of the Fishing Horse, T-Step). It is a comprehensive exercise for health, as are all the exercises in T'ai Chi.

QUESTION: What is the difference in exercising the sword and exercising with empty hands?**

ANSWER: The moment that you hold something in your hand, like a sword, a different situation exists, and this results in different conditions. You must contend with an object, and the space that you occupy has become larger. At the same time, the practice of letting go becomes quite clearly experienced when lowering the sword.

QUESTION: So, the sword as a weapon doesn't have a prominent place in practicing?

ANSWER: You could say that. Practicing the sword form, like practicing other forms, is first of all directed at the development of the ch'i. Think about the story of the master who fought with a meter-long tobacco pipe against the best sword fighter in China who held a sharp sword in his hand. The T'ai Chi master used sticking energy. He didn't need to hurt his opponent to win.

QUESTION: Is it possible to replace the sword with a different object if energy is developed?

ANSWER: Yes. We practice with dulled metal practice swords or with wooden swords. For many of the partner exercises, the wooden sword is even better suited than the metal practice sword. To improve yourself in the sword, and with it also

* With Petra Kobayashi, recorded by Beatrix Schumacher; first appeared in a German martial arts magazine in 1994 and translated in 2002 by Susan Rae Polzer.

** Expression for the short form and the long form in contrast to practicing the form with an object like a sword, a saber, or a staff.

in sword fighting, it is, therefore, insignificant if the sword is of metal or wood, if it is sharp or dull.

QUESTION: I've never seen a partner exercise with the sword. Is it comparable to the "Push Hands" in the other forms?

ANSWER: Yes. For example, there is a good partner exercise during which the application of the sticking energy is practiced. You walk through the room with the swords together and direct your sword with the techniques or free movements at the partner. But remember, the most important thing in the sword form is practicing for the development of the ch'i, also while working with a partner.

QUESTION: Is it wise, before one starts to practice the sword form, to learn the short form and the long form?

ANSWER: The sword form exists as an independent path. There are T'ai Chi sword masters who have never practiced with "empty hands." Nevertheless, as a rule, most practitioners first begin with the forms and then later add the sword.

QUESTION: Would you teach someone who has never practiced T'ai Chi but definitely only wanted to learn the sword form?

ANSWER: Yes. But this person would then need the same amount of time as in practicing the other forms to accomplish any deeper development.

QUESTION: Is practicing the sword form similar to a great extent to practicing the short form and the long form?

ANSWER: That's right, except for the things that we have already mentioned here. There is also a variation in the way of moving. Sometimes it is somewhat faster because the energy in the movement must be mobilized into the tip of the sword. As in the other forms, there is center equilibrium; the oneness of the body in movement; the guiding of the sword from the hips, that is, from the center; letting go, following, opening, and closing, and so on.

QUESTION: When does this similarity become clearer? Now, right at the beginning of my practicing the sword, I have the feeling, for example, that the little bit of lightness that I have acquired after practicing the forms for years is now lost again in the sword form. Perhaps it is simply because it is still foreign to me. How do you develop the perception that the sword is an extension of the arm, which is aimed for in the T'ai Chi sword?

ANSWER: It is purely a matter of practicing. Exercising with a sword trains the arm that holds the sword. So, it is not surprising that you first perceive the practicing to be strenuous. With time, it will become easier to hold the sword and to relax when performing the movements. To sense the sword as an extension of the arm is something that first occurs in advanced practicing and is explained in many ways through energy development. The energy then seizes or fills the sword, too—this is clearly felt by the practitioner.

QUESTION: Would a staff or another object also be filled with energy in the same manner?

ANSWER: Yes. At the same time, practicing leads to experiences of such a depth and fullness that reflections about the sword as a weapon become superficial. The energy development and perception lead into areas that are completely detached from labeling or naming, in sword fighting and self-defense, too. Something opens that is universal, that makes it completely unimportant what you have in your hand: a kitchen spoon, a tobacco pipe, or a sword. The more that this inner dimension of strengths and energies opens, the more that the "external" retreats. With it, the difference that many practitioners experienced in the beginning between the practicing of other forms and the sword forms ceases to be.

QUESTION: That is really interesting. The difference in the forms becomes relative, in a certain way, by itself through the inner development and perception that one gets.

ANSWER: I also wanted to say something else. Practicing with the sword trains one in body control and awareness in a special manner. We conduct ourselves in practicing sword as if the sword were sharp. In spite of all the things that I have said, this aspect, to be able to really fight with a sword, is of significance in our teaching.

QUESTION: Are all T'ai Chi masters also masters of the sword?

ANSWER: That can't be said. When you see the students of Cheng Man Ch'ing, the differences become clear. Only some of these teachers and masters are also experts in the sword. T. T. Liang was an exceptional sword fighter; he also learned the sword from the second generation of the Yang family. Others are also good, if only because they bring their energy development into the sword form, but they have less to do with the analysis of the techniques. For example, they teach the sword form without going into the techniques. That is also an expression of different interests.

QUESTION: What characterizes the Yang style sword forms?

ANSWER: The many sword forms in the Yang style draw upon the sword form handed down from Yang Cheng-Fu. It became widely known when it was recorded by Chen Wei-Ming, a student of Yang Cheng-Fu, who was also an important teacher. If one observes the many sword forms that have developed in the framework of the Yang style, then one finds that they follow the positions and normally the sequence given by Chen Wei-Ming, even when the transitions between the positions are handled differently.

QUESTION: What does the Cheng Man-Ch'ing sword form look like?

ANSWER: Cheng Man-Ch'ing also learned the sword form from Yang Cheng-Fu. Just as in his short form, in his sword form he has brought in his own special changes. For example, he emphasizes yielding through shifting backward in the transitions. The sword form taught by William Chen is quite similar.

QUESTION: Could someone who has no knowledge of T'ai Chi sword recognize it if he saw it?

ANSWER: An orientation for the beginner is basically difficult. It becomes more complicated because of the volume of the sword forms that are offered. The sword art tradition in China isn't only very old, but it is also exceptionally varied and widely distributed. This has led to many mixed forms, sword forms that contain elements from different martial arts including T'ai Chi Ch'uan. Many such forms that have reached the West are, nevertheless, offered as T'ai Chi sword forms. Moreover, they are frequently from teachers who have a different martial arts background than T'ai Chi and who bring their own distinctive way of moving and their own understanding of the techniques into the sword form.

QUESTION: Does the difference between the T'ai Chi sword forms and those of other martial arts exist because of its alignment with the principles of T'ai Chi Ch'uan?

ANSWER: Yes, and the principles come, on the other hand, from the Taoist background. They make the difference in the high art of the T'ai Chi sword, the exceptional refinement of the techniques. One can, or even better, one should, and even must, expect something special in a T'ai Chi sword form. This special quality can also be conveyed to the inexperienced spectator, provided that he is open to it. Sword forms, for example, where the sword is moved very rapidly without connection to the center of the body and only from the wrist have no T'ai Chi background. Unfortunately, it must be said here, that the T'ai Chi sword forms only open themselves to a farther-reaching understanding after a long period of learning and practicing. Also, in China, many of those interested are not prepared to take this path, and therein too lies the reason for the frequently observed watering down of the T'ai Chi sword forms. They don't have the patience to wait for the abilities that can only come through ch'i development and subscribe instead to methods that appear to be more effective and faster. But this changes the practicing and limits the development in the T'ai Chi Ch'uan sense.

QUESTION: This is an interesting and also far-reaching connection.

ANSWER: Yes. Therefore, it isn't easy, even in China, to find teachers with ch'i development in the sense of T'ai Chi Ch'uan and a well-grounded knowledge of T'ai Chi sword.

Glossary

CHEN, WILLIAM
A well-known T'ai Chi master in the United States, he was a student of Cheng Man-Ch'ing in Taiwan.

CHENG MAN-CH'ING (1900–1975)
Master of T'ai Chi, doctor, poet, and painter, he learned T'ai Chi Ch'uan from Yang Cheng-Fu. In the late forties, he went to Taiwan. In the sixties and seventies, he taught in the United States. Through the development of his short form, and through his books about T'ai Chi Ch'uan and Taoism, he influenced T'ai Chi Ch'uan in the West more than anyone else.

CHI CHIANG TAO (1920–1994)
Dr. Chi Chiang Tao was born in northern China in 1920. In 1937, he began his study of T'ai Chi Ch'uan because of a serious illness. He first learned the old Yang style from, among others, Tien Cheng-Feng. In 1948, he went to Taiwan and became a student of Cheng Man-Ch'ing. Today, he is still remembered as one of the best-known T'ai Chi masters in Taiwan and was a member of the Taiwan T'ai Chi Association, a union of students in the Cheng Man-Ch'ing tradition there. He was a master of T'ai Chi sword. In Taiwan, he practiced traditional Chinese medicine in addition to his teaching activities. In 1980, he moved to Vancouver, Canada.

CH'I
Cosmic or inner energy. (Japanese: Ki, Indian: Prana)

CHIN
The special abilities that result from the development and use of the ch'i that are understood to be separate energies; for example, t'ing chin (hearing energy), tung chin (interpreting energy), t'i chin (uprooting energy).

CHI KUNG
A collective term for mostly old Chinese exercises specifically applied for health that affect the activation of the ch'i.

CHANG SAN-FENG

Taoist master (end of the Sung Dynasty, 1127–1279), founder of the T'ai Chi Ch'uan from the Yang style point of view; known from the legends as a man of unusually large body size.

CLASSICAL TREATISES

Texts from the old masters in which the principles are written down. The most important ones are: Chang San-Feng, *The Classical Text of T'ai Chi Ch'uan*, Wang Tsung-Yueh, *The Theory of T'ai Chi Ch'uan*, Wu Yu-Hsiang, *The Practice of the Basic 13 Positions*.

FU ZHONG-WEN

Master Fu lived and taught in Shanghai; he was one of the outstanding students of Yang Cheng-Fu. He belonged to the few who didn't change Yang Cheng-Fu's form. He published a book on the long form of Yang Cheng-Fu, demonstrating the form in drawings based on existing photographs of Yang. This small book is a cult book on the Yang style in China. He managed the house of the Yang family, now a cultural site in Yongnian (northern China). His son, master Fu Shen-Yuan, lives and teaches in Australia.

HSING-I CH'UAN

"Mind boxing," founder uncertain, either: Yueh Fei (tenth century) or Chi Lung-Feng (seventeenth century). Hsing-I Ch'uan and Pa Kua belong to the "internal martial arts," as does T'ai Chi Ch'uan.

HSU

Sword master; the teacher of Dr. Chi; he learned among others, T'ai Chi sword from Wu Huei-Chuan, a well-known student of Yang Cheng-Fu; he learned San T'sai sword from Sun Lu-Tang and Chin Yun-Ting.

LIANG, T. T.

An exceptional T'ai Chi master in the Cheng Man-Ch'ing tradition, master of the sword who lived in the United States for a long time. He also taught partner exercises that were handed down from Yang Lu-Ch'an, which are similar to the San T'sai sword.

PA KUA

The "Boxing of the Eight Diagrams," origin unknown; first known master Tung Hai-Ch'uan (nineteenth century).

Push Hands (Tui Shou)
The most important partner exercise in the Yang style; based upon the basic positions of Ward Off, Roll Back, Press, and Push.

San T'sai sword
San T'sai (three treasures: heaven, earth, man); primarily contains partner exercises with a sword. It originated in northern China (Hopei Province). The first well-known teacher was Li Tsai-Te. San T'sai sword has a long family tradition.

Subtle energy realm
The entire subtle energy aspects, such as the meridian system, the subtle energy centers, aura, and so on.

Sun Lu-Tang (1861–1932)
Founder of the Sun style of T'ai Chi Ch'uan. His style contains elements of the Hsing-I-Ch'uan. Sun Lu-Tang was a close friend of Yang Cheng-Fu and General Li.

T'ai Chi Ch'uan
Putting together "T'ai Chi" and "Ch'uan." T'ai Chi = the mother of Yin and Yang, synonymous with the Tao; Ch'uan = hand or fist. The name T'ai Chi Ch'uan results logically: Through the hand or fist, in the method of the exercise, so as to be attuned with the Tao.

Tan t'ien
Lower, middle, and upper tan t'ien—the three tan t'iens belong to the most important subtle energy centers in the Taoist tradition.

Tao
The Ultimate, Nameless, the Mother of the myriad things.

Yang Cheng-Fu
Yang Cheng-Fu (1883–1936), third generation of the Yang family. His long form is the basis for the forms in the Yang style practiced today and for many other styles too, such as the Peking style.

Yang Lu-Ch'an
Founder of the Yang style (1799–1872).

YIN AND YANG

They represent all pairs of opposites. The alignment of T'ai Chi Ch'uan with the Yin and Yang demonstrates itself in the continuous changes in the movement from full to empty, weighted to unweighted, open to close, and so on.